Organ Transplants

Cathleen Small

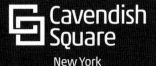

Cavendish
Square
New York

Published in 2019 by Cavendish Square Publishing, LLC
243 5th Avenue, Suite 136, New York, NY 10016

Library of Congress Cataloging-in-Publication Data

Names: Small, Cathleen, author.
Title: Organ transplants / Cathleen Small.
Description: First edition. | New York : Cavendish Square, 2019. | Series:
Great discoveries in science | Audience: Grades 9-12. | Includes
bibliographical references and index.
Identifiers: LCCN 2018010987 (print) | LCCN 2018012140 (ebook) | ISBN
9781502643698 (ebook) | ISBN 9781502643797 (library bound) |
ISBN 9781502643919 (pbk.)
Subjects: LCSH: Transplantation of organs, tissues, etc.—Juvenile literature.
Classification: LCC RD120.76 (ebook) | LCC RD120.76 .S63 2019 (print) | DDC 617.9/54—dc23
LC record available at https://lccn.loc.gov/2018010987

Editorial Director: David McNamara
Editor: Jodyanne Benson
Copy Editor: Michele Suchomel-Casey
Associate Art Director: Alan Sliwinski
Designer: Christina Shults
Production Coordinator: Karol Szymczuk
Photo Research: J8 Media

Printed in the United States of America

Contents

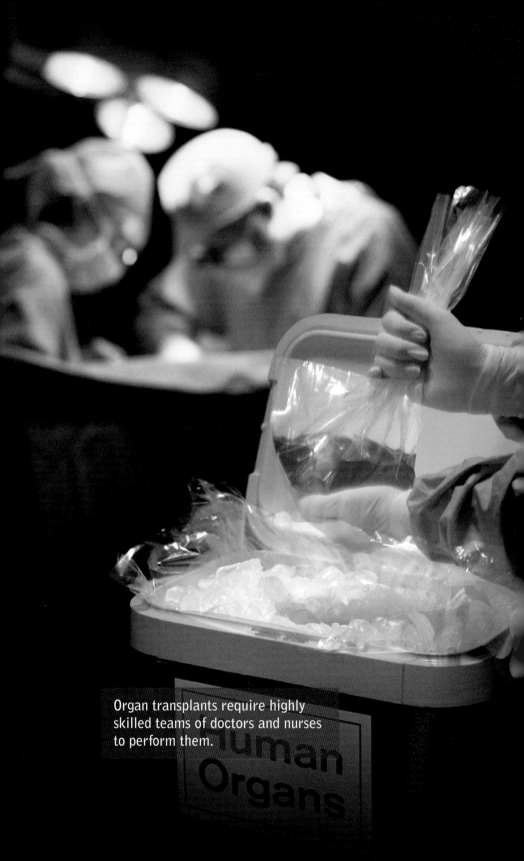

Organ transplants require highly skilled teams of doctors and nurses to perform them.

Introduction

Before organ transplantation became a viable treatment option, organ failure was essentially a death sentence for many patients. Some conditions, such as kidney failure, had temporary treatment options—dialysis, for example, can be used to keep a patient in kidney failure alive for a while. But it's a temporary solution—dialysis has far too many side effects to be a viable long-term solution. So, when organ transplants began to show real promise in the 1960s, it seemed like a near miracle for some people.

Still, as exciting as the technology is, and as much as it has saved many lives over the past decades, it's still not a perfect science or a permanent solution. Donated kidneys, for example, typically function from eight to twenty years, depending on whether they came from a live donor or a deceased donor. (Kidneys from a living donor typically last longer.) The survival rate for liver transplants is about five years. Heart recipients generally live somewhere between ten and twenty years, depending on a number of factors, with the longest-surviving heart recipient known to have lived for thirty-three years after his transplant.

Organ transplants in many cases buy time but not permanence. Some transplants, though, are not lifesaving, and so they buy quality of life more than anything else. For example, recipients of corneal transplants often weren't in any danger of death, but their quality of life greatly improved with the ability to see.

There's no doubt that the science of transplants has been beneficial and in many cases, lifesaving. But there is much development still to happen. As science progresses, particularly in fields like biotechnology and genetics, there are big developments looming on the horizon. Two big problems with organ transplants are organ rejection and an unequal supply and demand. Developments in science aim to tackle both of these problems.

Organ rejection is nearly guaranteed. The only time it doesn't occur is when the transplanted organ or tissue is genetically identical to the person who is receiving it. That happens when the transplant comes from one's own body (such as a skin graft with skin used from another part of the body) or if it comes from an identical twin. Otherwise, even if the donor and recipient are a good match, such as two members of the same family, organ rejection will happen if steps aren't taken to prevent it. It's simply how the immune system works. It sees a foreign tissue or organ in the body, and it attacks it. That's how the immune system fights off viruses and bacterial infections, and the same mechanism ends up fighting donor organs and tissues.

Scientists have developed immunosuppressant drugs to help combat this problem. However, the drugs have serious side effects, not the least of which is lowering the person's immune system overall, leaving him or her vulnerable to viruses and infections. Also, if a person forgets to take his or her immunosuppressants for even one day, it increases the chance of experiencing organ rejection. Immunosuppressants are a lifelong commitment after an organ transplant, which isn't a very appealing situation.

So, scientists are looking at ways to use technology to drastically reduce or potentially eliminate the need for immunosuppressants. Stem cells have shown a lot of promise in this area because they are undifferentiated cells that can be edited and can serve many functions.

Scientists have even experimented with growing new organs out of a recipient's own stem cells so that the organ will be genetically identical to the recipient. It's a very new technology and definitely not yet refined, but it's one way scientists are working to lower the rejection rates in organ transplantation.

Unequal supply and demand is another big problem with organ transplants. There are many more people who need transplants than there are donors. The waiting list is very long for organs, and every day people on the list die without having received a donor organ. Once again, scientists are looking at ways to potentially address this organ shortage.

One idea is to use stem cells to grow new organs, as mentioned earlier. Another idea is to use gene editing technology to breed animals that will have organs that can

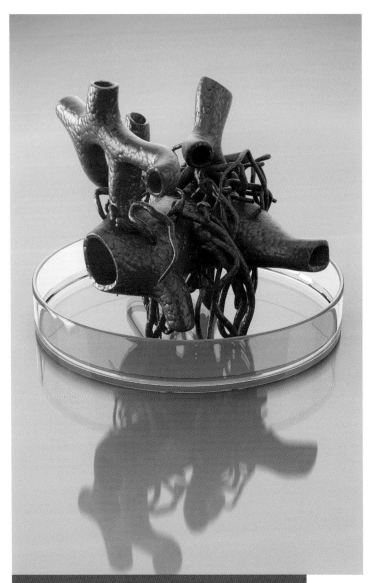

Bioprinting is a way to build models of tissue and organ structures. The circulatory system is shown here.

be transplanted to humans in need of transplant. Bioprinting is another solution. This technology enables living tissues, bones, blood vessels, and, potentially, whole organs to be used for teaching purposes and medical procedures.

Scientists are also looking at ways to make the best use of the organs that are available. For example, they are developing perfusion machines that work as sort of life-support devices for organs, to make donor organs last longer before transplant. This could enable a heart, for example, that becomes available on one coast to be flown to the opposite coast for transplant if that's where the best match for it is. Currently, with the use of cold-storage procedures, organs have a very limited life before they decay too much to be transplanted. So, a heart that becomes available on the West Coast, but has no recipient other than someone from the East Coast, will probably go to waste because there's no way to transport it that far before the organ becomes unusable. Technologies are being developed that can theoretically triple the lifespan of a donor organ.

While organ transplantation is something no one wants to have to face, it is an exciting time for the field, with new technologies and techniques improving outcomes all the time.

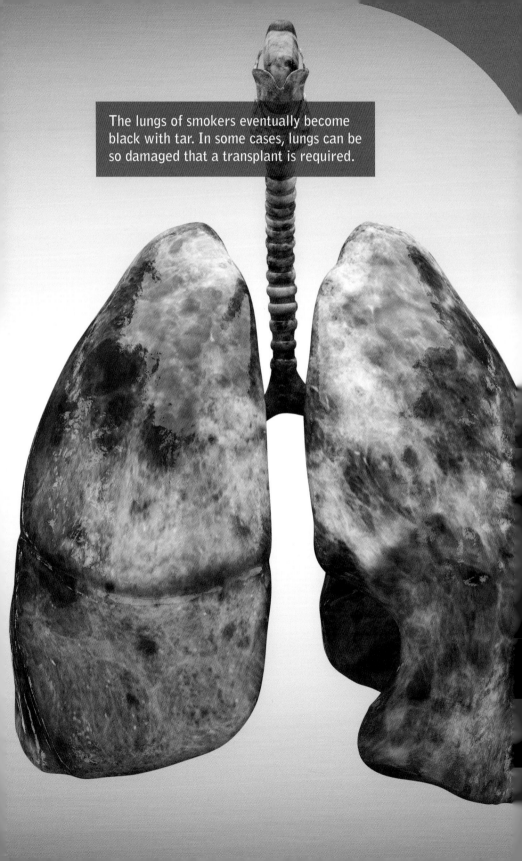

The lungs of smokers eventually become black with tar. In some cases, lungs can be so damaged that a transplant is required.

CHAPTER 1

The Problem of Organ Failure

O rgan transplantation is a relatively new science in the overall picture of human history. The first successful transplants took place in the 1950s, not even seventy years ago. But the idea of organ transplantation has been around for much longer because many of the problems that led to the development of successful transplants have been around since human life began. In much earlier generations, doctors may not have always known exactly what caused people to die, but in reality, the problem was the same general one that leads to transplants today: one or multiple organs become irreparably diseased or fail. Diseases change and develop over generations, but the end result doesn't change: diseases or chronic conditions harm body systems, and sometimes that harm ends in organ failure and can potentially be addressed with an organ transplant.

CAUSES of ORGAN FAILURE

According to the University of Michigan Transplant Center, in Ann Arbor, Michigan, there are a number of diseases and conditions that can cause organ failure and the need for a transplant. Organ failure can happen to the kidneys, liver, heart, lungs, or pancreas. The corneas can become damaged as well, which can be treated with a corneal transplant.

Causes of Kidney Failure

The conditions that most commonly cause kidney failure are diabetes, hypertensive nephrosclerosis, and glomerular disease.

Diabetes is a condition in which the pancreas cannot adequately produce insulin, which is necessary for metabolism. Diabetes can cause high levels of glucose in the bloodstream, which can damage the kidneys. It can also cause high blood pressure, which is damaging to the kidneys. This is why people with diabetes are at risk of kidney problems and sometimes kidney failure.

Diabetes has been around for thousands of years. Ancient Greek physician Aretaeus of Cappadocia first described it in the first century. Clearly, it has been causing organ failure since long before transplants were possible.

Another condition associated with diabetes and high blood pressure is nephrosclerosis, which is a hardening of the small blood vessels in the kidneys. It can lead to kidney failure.

Finally, kidney failure can be caused by glomerular diseases. Glomeruli are tiny units in the kidneys where blood is cleaned and then circulated out of the kidneys.

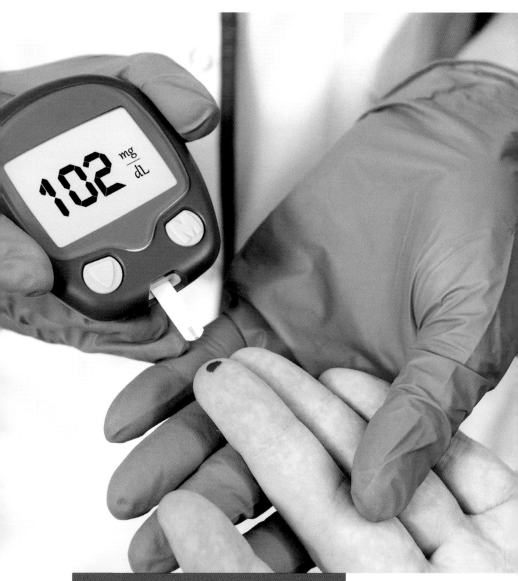

People with diabetes must monitor their glucose levels.

Glomerular diseases, which are diseases affecting the glomeruli, generally fall into two categories: glomerulonephritis and glomerulosclerosis.

Glomerulonephritis is when the membrane tissue in the kidneys that filters wastes and extra fluid from the blood becomes inflamed. Glomerulosclerosis is when the blood vessels in the kidneys become scarred and hardened.

Glomerular diseases can be caused by adverse drug reactions or by autoimmune diseases that attack the whole body, such as lupus or diabetes. They can also be caused as secondary responses to another infection, such as a streptococcal infection.

Causes of Liver Failure

Liver failure can result from many causes. Certain prescription medications and herbal supplements can cause it, as can an overdose of acetaminophen (commonly known in the United States as Tylenol).

Several types of hepatitis can also lead to liver failure, including hepatitis A, B, and E. Hepatitis is an inflammation of the liver that can result from a number of causes. Hepatitis A is the result of a virus spread by eating contaminated food or drinking contaminated water. Hepatitis B is also caused by a virus, but it is transmitted by exposure to infected bodily fluids, such as blood. Like hepatitis A, hepatitis E is caused by a virus and spreads by ingesting contaminated food or water.

All these variants of hepatitis can lead to cirrhosis, which is scarring of the liver. Hepatitis attacks the liver, and when the liver tries to repair itself, scar tissue forms. Cirrhosis can also be caused by alcohol abuse, autoimmune diseases such as autoimmune hepatitis, and accumulation of fat in the liver. There are a handful of other conditions that can lead to cirrhosis as well, but not as commonly as hepatitis, alcohol abuse, autoimmune disease, or fatty liver.

Liver failure can also be a result of sepsis, cancer, or certain rare metabolic diseases. Sepsis is the result of an infection somewhere in the body that causes the body's immune response to attack the body's own tissues and organs. Usually, the infection is bacterial, but sometimes it's caused

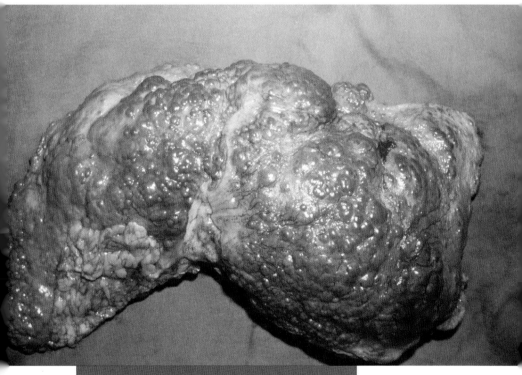

This unhealthy liver has been attacked by cirrhosis, a major cause of liver failure.

by a virus, parasite, or fungus. Typically, the body can handle infections like these without complication, but in people with weaker immune systems (due to age or conditions that result in weakened immune systems, such as cancer), sepsis is a concern. Sepsis can be treated successfully and doesn't always lead to organ failure. When it's caught early, sepsis has a recovery rate of approximately 70 percent. But if sepsis is ignored or if the person's body doesn't respond to treatment, sepsis can become severe and ultimately result in organ failure.

Sepsis has been around for many generations. Greek physician Hippocrates (460–370 BCE) even discussed sepsis. And the World Health Organization (WHO) has called hepatitis A one of the oldest diseases known to humankind. Clearly, then, at least two causes of liver failure have been around for thousands of years, long before organ transplantation was a treatment option.

Causes of Heart Failure

The conditions that most commonly cause heart failure are coronary artery disease, high blood pressure, faulty heart valves, cardiomyopathy, myocarditis, arrhythmia, and congenital heart defects.

Coronary heart disease is the most common cause for heart failure. This disease results when fatty plaque deposits form in the arteries, which reduces blood flow. These plaque deposits can form when a person has too much bad cholesterol in his or her system. (There are good and bad cholesterols; low-density lipoproteins, or LDLs, are generally referred to as bad cholesterols, whereas high-density lipoproteins, or HDLs, are generally referred to as good cholesterols.)

Just as high blood pressure can damage the kidneys, so too can it damage the heart. It forces the heart to work harder than usual to pump blood, which can weaken or stiffen the heart muscle.

Heart valves help move blood through the heart. If one is faulty, due to coronary artery disease, an infection, or a heart defect, it has to work harder to pump blood, and as with high blood pressure, this can ultimately weaken the heart muscle.

Cardiomyopathy refers to a condition in which the heart muscle is damaged. It can be caused by disease, infection, adverse reactions to certain drugs (such as those used for chemotherapy), use of certain illegal drugs, or alcohol abuse.

Myocarditis, an inflammation of the heart, is most often caused by a virus, bacteria, parasite, or fungus. It can also (less commonly) be caused by adverse drug reactions, use of certain illegal drugs, exposure to certain chemicals or radiation, and a few rare diseases. Myocarditis can lead to failure of the left side of the heart.

Arrhythmia refers to abnormal heart rhythms. Many arrhythmias can be benign, but sometimes arrhythmias can cause the heart to have to work harder and can lead to heart failure.

Finally, congenital heart defects refer to problems with the formation of the heart. Some people are born with these defects, and often they can be corrected through surgery. But they can also cause the heart to have to work harder than usual, which can lead to heart failure.

Some of these causes of heart failure are relatively recent developments, such as cardiomyopathy or myocarditis resulting from the use of certain drugs or exposure to radiation. But some of these causes, such as congenital heart defects and infections or inflammations due to viruses or bacteria, have been around for thousands of years.

Causes of Respiratory Failure

Lung failure, commonly called respiratory failure, can be caused by cystic fibrosis, pulmonary fibrosis, pulmonary hypertension, sarcoidosis, emphysema, or chronic obstructive pulmonary disease.

Cystic fibrosis (CF) is an inherited condition that some people are born with. A gene mutation causes secretions of mucus, which are normally thin, to become very sticky and thick. This mucus then clogs the tubes, ducts, and passages in the lungs and sometimes the pancreas. It is a fatal condition that most often can be treated but not cured. However, lung transplants do increase the chance of long-term survival greatly because CF does not reoccur in transplanted lungs. (It can, however, continue to harm other organs in the body.)

Pulmonary fibrosis occurs when lung tissue becomes thickened or scarred. This can occur from many causes, and sometimes there is no apparent cause. But in cases where the cause can be determined, pulmonary fibrosis can result from environmental factors, such as exposure to certain types of dust or toxins, damage from radiation treatments, damage from certain medications, infections such as pneumonia, and some autoimmune conditions, such as lupus and rheumatoid arthritis.

Pulmonary hypertension is a specific type of high blood pressure that affects the right side of the heart and the arteries in the lungs. The pulmonary arterioles, which are tiny arteries in the lungs, can become blocked, narrowed, or destroyed, raising the pressure inside the larger arteries in the lungs and forcing the heart and lungs to work harder, which can ultimately result in organ failure.

There are five types of pulmonary hypertension that result from many causes, including heart disease or defect, blood disorders and clots, metabolic disorders, gene mutations, chronic conditions such as lupus or cirrhosis, and even sleep apnea.

Sarcoidosis is a condition in which granulomas form in different areas in the body as the result of an immune response. No exact cause has yet been pinpointed for sarcoidosis, but so far it appears that some people are genetically predisposed to develop it. It can be triggered by dust, chemicals, bacteria, or viruses.

In people with emphysema, the alveoli in the lungs get weakened and rupture, which creates fewer large air sacs, rather than many smaller air sacs. This, in turn, reduces the amount of oxygen that reaches the person's bloodstream because the surface area of the lungs is decreased. Emphysema is most often caused by smoke from tobacco products or marijuana, but it can also be caused by air pollution or chemical fumes and dust.

Emphysema is one type of chronic obstructive pulmonary disease (COPD), which is another major cause

Cystic Fibrosis

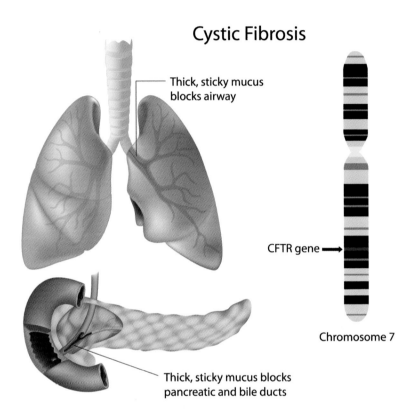

Thick, sticky mucus blocks airway

CFTR gene ➞

Chromosome 7

Thick, sticky mucus blocks pancreatic and bile ducts

A double-lung transplant can greatly increase the lifespan of someone suffering from cystic fibrosis.

of respiratory failure. COPD is a chronic inflammatory lung disease that is most often caused by smoking tobacco products. Rarely, COPD is the result of a genetic disorder called alpha-1-antitrypsin deficiency. That results for only about 1 percent of all COPD cases; exposure to smoke or other chemicals is the far more common cause.

Just as with the causes of heart failure, some of these causes of respiratory failure are relatively recent. Exposure to toxic chemicals leading to emphysema, for example, is a relatively recent development in the history of humankind. But other causes for respiratory failure have undoubtedly been around for much longer. Although cystic fibrosis wasn't officially diagnosed until the 1930s, it's thought to have been noted as early as the 1700s, for example.

Causes of Pancreatic Failure

Failure of the pancreas is often the result of diabetes, but cancers of the pancreas or bile duct can also result in failure of the pancreas.

There are two types of diabetes: type 1 and type 2. Type 1 diabetes is a condition in which the pancreas produces little to no insulin. It is an autoimmune condition that is often also called insulin-dependent diabetes or juvenile diabetes.

Type 2 diabetes is often called adult-onset diabetes or noninsulin-dependent diabetes. In type 2 diabetes, the body either doesn't produce enough insulin or resists the effects of insulin.

While type 1 diabetes requires people to inject insulin for the rest of their lives, type 2 diabetes can often be treated with healthy lifestyle choices, such as losing weight, getting enough exercise, and making healthy food choices.

Pancreas transplants usually only work for people with type 1 diabetes. They aren't typically done for people with type 2 diabetes or pancreatic cancer because these conditions usually cannot be treated effectively with a transplant. Even in type 1 diabetes, transplants aren't common because the side effects can be serious.

Diabetes is an incredibly old condition. It was first mentioned by Hesy-Ra, an Egyptian physician, in 1552 BCE. Clearly, it was around long before organ transplantation became an option!

Causes of Corneal Damage

Corneal transplants are an option when a person's corneas become damaged or diseased, which can lead to loss of vision. Corneal damage and disease can be the result of keratoconus, certain degenerative conditions, corneal perforations, corneal scars, or resistant infections in the cornea.

Keratoconus causes the cornea to thin, change shape, and weaken. It's unclear exactly what causes it, but it's more common in people with allergic conditions such as asthma and eczema. Keratoconus can be a mild condition, but if it gets severe, a corneal transplant may be the best treatment.

There are certain degenerative conditions, such as Fuchs endothelial dystrophy, that can cause damage to the cornea. In this condition, the cells that line the inner cornea begin to deteriorate, causing extra fluid to build up in the eyes. This results in cloudy vision.

Corneal perforations are small holes in the cornea that can happen if the eye is damaged. Corneal scars also occur from damage, but they can form if a person has a corneal infection.

Many corneal infections can be treated with antibiotics, but in the case of an infection that persists despite treatment with antibiotics, a corneal transplant may eventually be required.

Causes of Multiple Organ Failure

Multiple organ failure, which is when more than one organ fails at generally the same time, is often the result of sepsis or systemic inflammatory response syndrome (SIRS). There are other conditions that can cause it as well, such as acute pancreatitis, but in general, it is often caused by sepsis or SIRS.

Unlike sepsis, SIRS is a relatively new diagnosis. Dr. William Nelson at the University of Toronto, in Ontario, Canada, first discussed the condition in 1983. SIRS refers to systemic inflammation in the body that may or may not be caused by infection. SIRS can be caused by trauma, burns, pancreatitis, ischemia, or hemorrhage. SIRS can lead to sepsis in some cases, but sometimes it is simply SIRS that causes organs to begin to fail.

Fibrosis is a condition that can also lead to organ failure, especially heart or kidney failure. Fibrosis occurs when the body forms excess connective tissue, which causes scarring on organ tissues. It can affect the lungs, liver, heart, brain, digestive system, joints, bone marrow, skin, and soft tissues.

Face Transplants

Face transplants are a relatively new entry into the transplant field, with the United States being one of the leading countries in face transplant research. They aren't terribly common; it's much more common for patients to have facial reconstruction, which involves using skin from other parts of the patient's body to perform a series of surgeries designed to patch back together the person's face. In a few severe cases, a face "replant" has been successfully performed. The first of such a surgery was in 1994, when a young girl in India had her face completely ripped off into two pieces by getting her hair caught in a threshing machine. The two pieces of her face were brought to the hospital in a plastic bag, and surgeons were able to reattach them, although the young girl does have permanent scarring and muscle damage.

In some cases of people seriously disfigured by burns, birth defects, disease, or trauma, a face transplant may be the most viable solution. In 2005, a French woman was mauled by her dog, and surgeons grafted the nose and mouth from a brain-dead person onto the patient. This marked the first successful partial face transplant in history.

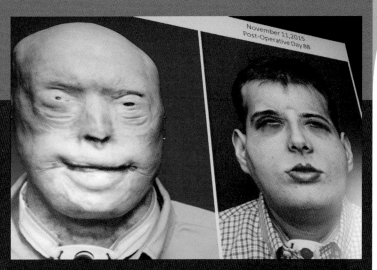

November 11,2015
Post-Operative Day 88

This extensive face transplant, which took place in New York City, took more than twenty-four hours to complete. The recipient was a volunteer firefighter who had sustained extensive burns to his face.

Research continues in face transplants, especially in the United States, Turkey, France, and Spain. Face transplants are incredibly complicated, involving not only skin but also nerves, blood vessels, and sometimes fat, bones, and muscles. The surgery typically takes anywhere between eight and thirty-six hours, and patients remain in the hospital for up to two weeks. So far, only four patients have died as a result of complications stemming from face transplants.

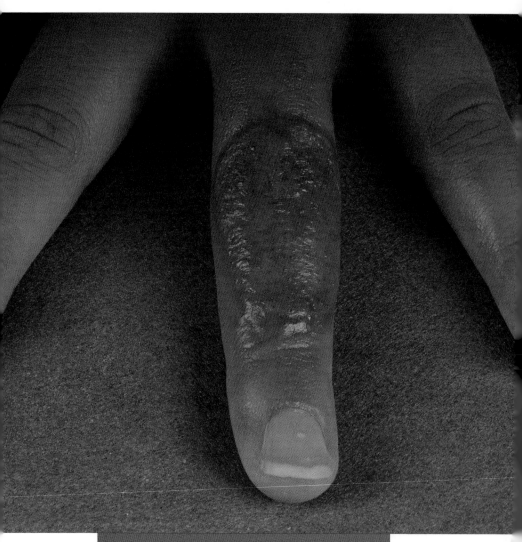

Skin grafts have been successfully performed for quite some time. One reason why is that skin can often be used from another area on the patient's own body.

Fibrosis can be caused by injury. Basically, it's the formation of scar tissue. However, in the absence of injury or inflammation, it is also thought to be caused by two proteins in the body, transforming growth factor beta 1 (also called TGF-β1) and interleukin-11 (known as IL-11). Scientists have long been working on ways to inhibit production of TGF-β1, but the current treatment has some severe side effects. The rule of IL-11 in fibrosis is a more recent discovery, and scientists hope to find ways to inhibit the protein, thereby slowing or stopping the progression of fibrosis. But until these treatments have been perfected, people around the world suffer from fibrosis and sometimes organ failure. A recent study reported that, as of 2017, more than 225 million people globally were suffering from heart and kidney failure.

While it's impossible to know whether people in past generations suffered from fibrosis, it's likely the condition has been around for a very long time and has been causing organ failure for many generations.

EARLY INTEREST in ORGAN TRANSPLANTATION

Clearly, there has been a need for organ transplants since very early in the history of humankind. The first successful transplant of an organ, other than a cornea, wasn't done until 1954, but there was interest long before then. Legend suggests that Bian Que, the first known Chinese physician, who died in 310 BCE, performed a heart transplant between two men, though that legend is unproven. In 2008, the *Journal of the Balkan Union of Oncology* published a piece about Roman Catholic saints Cosmas and Damian, who supposedly transplanted the leg of a deceased Moor onto a Roman deacon who lived from 527–565 CE. That account is also unproven.

While these two earliest mentions are highly questionable, there is decent evidence to suggest that early skin transplants, or grafts, were successful. Sushruta, an Indian surgeon who lived in the sixth century BCE, reportedly performed a skin graft while reconstructing a patient's nose. Sixteenth-century Italian surgeon Gasparo Tagliacozzi was reportedly successful with skin grafts and was considered a pioneer of reconstructive surgery.

In the 1700s, scientists performed experiments with organ transplants on animals and humans, and in 1837, researchers successfully transplanted a cornea in a gazelle model. Just over fifty years later, Dr. Theodor Kocher, who later won a Nobel Prize, performed the first successful thyroid transplant. Kocher's work prompted important research and experimentation with transplants around the early twentieth century.

One such example is French surgeon Alexis Carrel, who, along with Dr. Charles Guthrie, pioneered surgical techniques used in the transplantation of arteries and veins. Carrel also experimented with transplantation in dogs and ultimately discovered the problem of organ rejection. Carrel's pioneering work in the field earned him the 1912 Nobel Prize in Physiology or Medicine.

After World War I, research into organ transplantation slowed drastically, when scientists could not determine a good solution for the problems raised by organ rejection. The exception was work with skin grafts, which continued and, in fact, progressed significantly during World War I. This progress occurred in large part because of the work of Harold Gillies, a London-based head and neck surgeon who is also considered one of the fathers of modern plastic surgery.

In 1933, Ukrainian surgeon Yurii Voronoy attempted the first kidney transplant from a deceased human donor, but it failed due to problems with the blood vessels. After that, studies in organ rejection, immunosuppressive drugs, and tissue-typing helped make future attempts at organ transplant much more successful.

We will now explore the science behind the discovery of organ transplantation. By examining the work of the pioneers in the field, we will learn about how researchers, doctors, and scientists build on knowledge and discoveries of the past in order to solve today's problems.

INTERNAL STRUCTURE OF THE HUMAN BODY

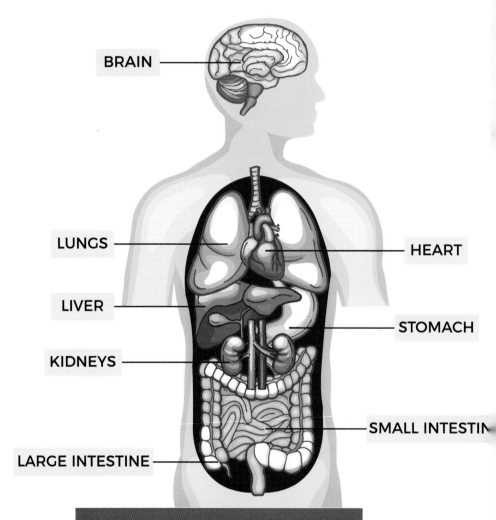

BRAIN

LUNGS

LIVER

KIDNEYS

LARGE INTESTINE

HEART

STOMACH

SMALL INTESTIN

Most major organs in the body can now be
transplanted—except the brain.

CHAPTER 2

The Science of Organ Transplants

S cience is an ever-evolving field, and later discoveries build on knowledge gained from earlier experiments and hypotheses. Part of why organ transplant is such a relatively new field is that scientists and the medical community had to learn a lot about how the body is formed and how it functions before they could even begin to think about transplanting organs.

BREAKING DOWN the BODY

There's a hierarchy of structures that lead up to a human body. The smallest unit of a chemical element is an atom. Atoms make up molecules. One type of molecule is a nucleotide. Nucleotides join together to form DNA, which carries the unique genetic code of each individual. DNA is found on chromosomes, which exist in the nucleus of most living cells.

It's critically important for scientists to understand DNA, chromosomes, and genetics in order to understand a great number of conditions that can lead to health complications in people. Some people need organ transplants for reasons that may have nothing to do with genetics. For example, people who abuse alcohol for an extended period of time may do damage to their liver that ultimately results in the need for a transplant. Or, a perfectly healthy person could contract a virus that leads to a complication that weakens the heart, ultimately requiring a heart transplant.

But in many cases, there is a genetic component to conditions that cause people to require transplants. For example, both type 1 and type 2 diabetes have been linked to genetic factors. They're not always caused by genetics, but there are at least five genetic mutations that have been identified as increasing a person's risk of developing type 2 diabetes and at least three genetic mutations that have been identified as increasing a person's risk of developing type 1 diabetes.

Diabetics sometimes end up needing organ transplants. They usually need kidney transplants because of the damage diabetes can do to their kidneys. One might think that a pancreas transplant would be needed since diabetes is a result of the pancreas not effectively producing insulin. But in studying how diabetes works and the effects the two types have on the pancreas, scientists have learned that pancreas transplants are not an effective treatment for type 2 diabetics.

DISEASE and IMMUNOLOGY

For similar reasons, it was important for scientists to develop a strong body of knowledge about disease and immunology. Certain diseases attack organs, but whether a transplant is the best course of treatment depends on the disease and how it functions. For example, pancreatic cancer is a particularly devastating diagnosis because the survival rate from chemotherapy or other treatments is quite low. For patients with exocrine pancreatic cancer, the five-year survival rate is at most 12 percent. It can be as low as 1 percent, depending on the stage at which the cancer is diagnosed. However, by studying pancreatic cancer and how it functions in the body, scientists have learned that pancreas transplants are not an effective treatment because the cancer has a high likelihood of metastasizing and attacking the new pancreas.

One might wonder what the harm is in at least trying a pancreas transplant in a person dying of pancreatic cancer. More than anything, it's a supply-and-demand issue. There are far more people waiting for organs than there are available organs. It's not uncommon for people on the organ transplant list (for nearly any organ) to die before a matching organ is found. So, it makes sense to perform pancreas transplants for patients in which the procedure is likely to be successful. Pancreatic cancer moves so swiftly that the longer a person waits for a pancreas to become available, the more advanced the cancer will be and the greater the likelihood that it will recur and claim the person's life quickly. While it sounds harsh to make a judgment call on who is more deserving of an available organ, from a purely objective standpoint, it makes sense to use the few organs that are available for the patients that are the most likely to benefit from them for the long term.

One frequent cause of organ damage is autoimmune diseases. There are more than one hundred known autoimmune diseases that affect all different parts of the body, but they all have something in common: they involve the body attacking itself. Basically, when a person suffers from an autoimmune disease, his or her body mistakes normal body cells for foreign cells and mounts an immune response. The immune system releases antibodies that attack the cells the body thinks are foreign.

Some autoimmune diseases attack a single organ. Type 1 diabetes, for example, attacks the pancreas. (Kidney damage is a side effect of type 1 diabetes; the immune system doesn't directly attack the kidneys.) But other autoimmune diseases, such as multiple sclerosis and lupus, attack multiple parts of the body or the whole body.

Understanding how autoimmune diseases work has been essential to scientists who work in the field of organ transplant. For example, by understanding how type 1 and type 2 diabetes function, scientists have learned that pancreas transplants can successfully cure type 1 diabetes, but they are not an effective treatment for type 2 diabetes. In type 1 diabetes, the pancreas has failed, and so replacing it with a transplanted organ may solve the problem. (However, pancreas transplants are not common because the side effects can be severe, and for most type 1 diabetics, a safer course of treatment is to monitor blood glucose throughout the day and give self-injections multiple times a day to regulate the amount of insulin in the body.)

In type 2 diabetes, however, the problem is not with the pancreas failing; rather, the issue is that the body has become unable to use insulin properly. So, the failure is with the body, not with the pancreas itself, and thus even with a transplanted pancreas, the body wouldn't know how to use the insulin the organ would produce.

Understanding autoimmune diseases that attack the entire body has given scientists insight into which ones make a person a good candidate for a transplant and which don't. Multiple sclerosis, for example, damages the central nervous system. Since nerves handle communication from the brain to every part of the body, multiple sclerosis eventually attacks the entire body. People with multiple sclerosis are not good candidates for organ transplants because even if an organ is failing due to complications from the disease, the new organ would simply suffer from the same fate. There's no way, at least right now, to transplant the central nervous system, and that would be the only way to truly cure the disease.

Interestingly, though, people with multiple sclerosis can donate organs. They cannot donate blood or bone marrow, but they can donate their other organs. Whether those organs will be used is determined on a case-by-case basis by the medical team, but there is nothing preventing a person with multiple sclerosis from trying to donate his or her organs.

The reason why blood and marrow transplants aren't allowed is because the exact cause of multiple sclerosis is unknown, and people receiving transfusions of either don't know anything about the donor. Thus, the patient cannot make an informed decision about whether to accept the blood or marrow. With organs, people can be given basic information about who the organ came from and can then make an informed decision about whether to accept the risk of an organ from a donor with multiple sclerosis or whether to turn down the organ and remain on the transplant list until an organ from a healthy person becomes available.

Lupus is another autoimmune disease that attacks multiple parts of the body, but some patients with lupus can get organ transplants. In fact, kidney transplants are regularly done on patients with lupus since lupus attacks the kidneys in 60 percent of patients with the autoimmune disease. In late 2017, lupus got much attention in the press when pop star Selena Gomez, then twenty-five years old, got a kidney transplant because of damage to her kidneys from lupus.

The risk-benefit scenario for kidney transplants in lupus patients is highly positive. Doctors and scientists have found that patients with lupus who have related kidney disease typically live longer if they have a kidney transplant than they do if they have long-term dialysis. Research has shown that lupus rarely recurs in a transplanted kidney.

CELL DIVISION, REPRODUCTION, and ORGAN DEVELOPMENT

Clearly, understanding how genetics, diseases, and immunology function in the body is critical to learning when organ transplantation is likely to be successful and when it's not. But there was more scientific knowledge necessary for scientists to eventually arrive at the discovery of organ transplants. Scientists needed to understand how cells reproduce in the body and how organs are developed and begin to function in the body.

Babies do not have organs when the embryo is first developing. When an egg is initially fertilized by a sperm cell, the fertilized egg has one thing that makes it able to develop into a person: the genetic material that contains the

Fertilized Cell Development

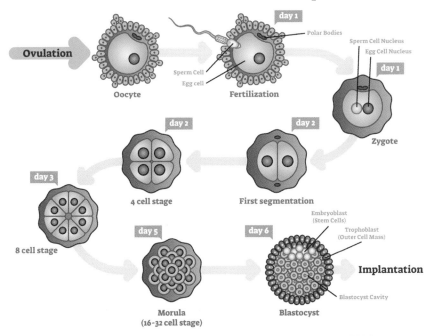

Ovulation

Oocyte

Sperm Cell

Egg cell

Fertilization

day 1

Polar Bodies

Sperm Cell Nucleus

Egg Cell Nucleus

day 1

Zygote

day 2

day 2

First segmentation

4 cell stage

day 3

8 cell stage

day 5

Morula
(16-32 cell stage)

day 6

Embryoblast
(Stem Cells)

Trophoblast
(Outer Cell Mass)

Blastocyst

Blastocyst Cavity

Implantation

The earliest stages of human development occur in the days following fertilization of an egg.

blueprint for how the person will form. As mentioned, that genetic information is stored in DNA, which is found on chromosomes. Humans typically have twenty-three pairs of chromosomes. (Certain chromosomal conditions, such as Down syndrome, alter this number of chromosomes. But most people have twenty-three pairs, for a total of forty-six chromosomes.) In a fertilized egg, also called a zygote, one chromosome in each pair has been donated by the sperm cell, and the other chromosome in each pair was present in the egg. Eggs and sperm cells are the only cells in the human body that contain only half the usual

Theodor Kocher: Transplant Pioneer

In science, sometimes the most important people are the ones who discover something that leads to other major discoveries. Such is the case with Theodor Kocher, a Nobel Prize–winning Swiss surgeon who was well regarded for his contributions

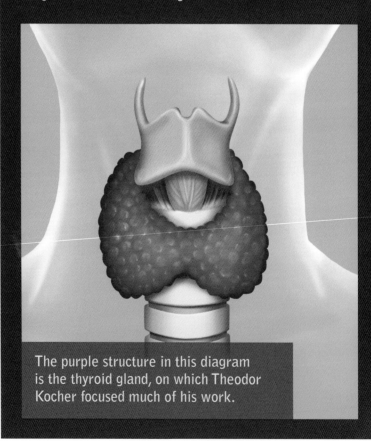

The purple structure in this diagram is the thyroid gland, on which Theodor Kocher focused much of his work.

to the development of aseptic surgery techniques and his contributions to the field of neurosurgery and epilepsy.

But it was Kocher's work in thyroid surgery that led him to make an important contribution to the field of organ transplantation. Kocher was an accomplished thyroid surgeon. In the 1870s, when Kocher began performing these surgeries, the mortality rate for complete removal of the thyroid was approximately 75 percent. Using surgical precision and aseptic techniques, Kocher helped drastically reduce the mortality rate.

However, Kocher then discovered that complete thyroidectomy sometimes led to cretinism, a condition with severe physical and mental side effects. In 1883, he began implanting human thyroid tissue to see whether it would correct the loss of thyroid hormone from the thyroidectomy. The experiment worked, and it is considered the first successful non-skin-tissue transplant.

number of chromosomes, and that is because each donates chromosomes to create a newly developing human with the typical forty-six chromosomes (or twenty-three pairs).

Immediately after fertilization, the single-cell zygote begins to divide into a mass of cells, called a blastocyst. In the earliest stages of development, the cells are nondifferentiated. They are stem cells that haven't become differentiated cells with specific functions, such as blood cells, skin cells, or nerve cells. Once the blastocyst has implanted into the uterine wall (usually several days after fertilization), the cells begin to replicate more rapidly, and cells begin to differentiate into specific cell types.

This is important for two reasons. First, in recent years stem cells have been found to be incredibly promising for treating certain diseases and conditions, and they are even showing promise in terms of growing new organs. Because stem cells are undifferentiated, they can do anything— they're sort of jack-of-all-trades cells. Stem cell transplants are becoming an increasingly common treatment for cancers like leukemia and lymphoma, as well as for certain blood diseases. While adults do have some stem cells in their bodies, scientists have learned that stem cells from adults are in short supply and don't tend to be as usable as embryonic stem cells.

Second, the process of fertilization and embryonic development has been important for scientists because the point at which an embryo is implanted and starts to develop into differentiated cells is the point at which organs are at the very first stages of forming. Understanding how organs form is key to understanding how in the future, stem cells might be used to grow new organs to be used in transplants.

Scientists are already experimenting with this technology. They've grown several organs using animal stem cells in labs, and in 2016, scientists from Massachusetts General Hospital and Harvard Medical School, both in Boston, revealed that they had successfully created a beating human heart by turning adult skin cells into stem cells and then inducing those stem cells to become cardiac cells.

Research like this could be monumental for the field of organ transplantation. One of the biggest risks to organ transplants is rejection. If scientists can learn how to use stem cells to grow new organs from a person's own cells, in theory that organ could be transplanted into the person without risk of rejection.

Research teaches scientists many things. One thing scientists working in this particular field have found is that organs grow best with a particular scaffolding. In a typically developing embryo and fetus, organs don't grow completely separately, with no scaffolding.

The initial ball of cells is the scaffolding on which all of the organs begin to form. It's like the architecture and subsequent building of a house. The genetic code in the zygote is like the architect's blueprint for a house, and the initial ball of cells is like the frame of the house. Once the house is framed, the different rooms can be divided, the plumbing and electrical can be installed, and slowly the house comes together into one whole.

The same is true with a developing embryo and fetus. Once the "framing" of the ball of cells is there and certain organs begin to develop, then other organs have a scaffolding on which to develop. Eventually, the fetus comes together as a functioning whole, with all organs working together.

Knowing this, the Massachusetts General Hospital and Harvard scientists who grew the beating heart took seventy-three donor hearts (all of which had been deemed unfit for transplant) and stripped them of cells that would set off an immune response. They then used the stripped heart "frames" and placed the stem cells they had turned into cardiac cells into those frames. The stem-cells-turned-cardiac-cells then grew into a functioning heart on the frame of another heart.

This incredible development would not have been possible if scientists had not done much research over many generations to learn how organs form and grow in a developing embryo and fetus.

BRAIN DEATH and ORGAN HARVEST

Organs are donated in two main ways. In a living-donor situation, a living person is donating an organ or a part of an organ that he or she can live without. For example, people can live with only one kidney, so it's not uncommon for a relative to donate a kidney to a family member who needs one. The liver is the only organ in the body that can regenerate itself (other than the skin, which frequently regenerates to repair injuries), so living-donor liver transplants aren't uncommon. Living-donor lung and pancreas transplants are becoming more common, too, since people can live without pieces of those organs.

The second way in which organs are donated is when a person dies, either by brain death or cardiac death. Cardiac death is what it sounds like: the heart stops beating and the circulatory system stops. Brain death isn't always

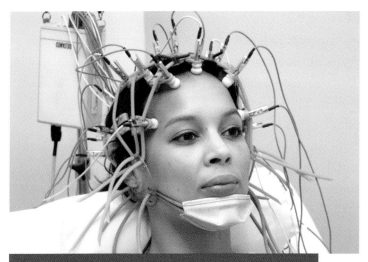

Brain death can be assessed by an **EEG**, which measures electrical activity in the brain.

technically death. In fact, its definition is somewhat inconsistent. Technically, it means that the person has suffered irreversible loss of all brain functions, including those vital functions controlled by the brain stem, such as reflexes and breathing.

However, some people consider brain death to be synonymous with a persistent vegetative state that never resolves, in which the patient will never regain consciousness and most of his or her brain functioning is irreversibly lost. The patient's basic vital functions, however, may still be somewhat intact. People in this state can be kept alive indefinitely on life support, and so it sometimes becomes an ethical or legal question as to whether the person should be kept alive or whether they should be taken off life support and potentially have their organs donated. (In an ideal world, all people would legally document their wishes if they were to ever end up in this state, but in reality, many people have not prepared an advance directive, and it is then up to their families to make decisions about care and removal of life support.)

Brain death, then, can be a complicated issue. However, laws are in place to make it as objective as possible. A physician doesn't simply assess a patient and determine he or she is brain dead. Many tests are done on the patient to determine what parts, if any, of the brain are still functioning. Gag, pupil, and breathing reflexes are checked, among other factors. Usually, if the brain-stem functions and/or circulatory and respiratory functions have ceased irreversibly, the patient can be declared brain dead. At that point, either the patient's advance directive can be followed or the family can decide whether to remove life support and potentially release the person's organs for donation.

When an organ comes from a deceased donor, medical teams know how to determine whether the organ is usable and who might be a suitable recipient for it. They know how to do this based on the exhaustive research and experimentation scientists have done to determine how long organs can survive after cardiac or brain death and how to tissue-type the organ.

In cardiac death, the heart and circulation have stopped. Because most organs need blood circulation to survive, the vital organs such as the heart, kidney, liver, and lungs very quickly become unusable. However, certain parts of the body can be harvested for donation for up to twenty-four hours, including skin, heart valves, and corneas.

There is also an exception to this: sometimes cardiac death occurs because a person is taken off life support. The person may have nonrecoverable injuries but still have some brain-stem function, so he or she is able to survive on a ventilator. If the person has an advance directive specifying he or she is not to be kept alive by artificial means or if the family makes that decision in lieu of an advance directive, the ventilator can be removed in an operating room.

When the heart stops beating on its own, cardiac death has occurred, and surgeons can immediately remove the organs for transplant. Because of the very short usability window of vital organs after cardiac death, the transplant has to happen pretty much immediately. This is why people who die naturally of something like a heart attack are not able to be organ donors for vital organs. Too much time elapses between the heart stopping and the organs being removed.

ORGAN PLACEMENT

Before organ donation could become a reality, scientists also had to learn how to match potential donors and recipients. Not everyone can receive any person's organ; certain factors need to match for there to be a chance of success.

The first factor is blood type. Donors and recipients must have compatible blood types. The blood types are A, AB, B, and O. O is the universal donor, which means that any person can receive an organ from a donor who has blood type O. However, recipients with type O can receive an organ only from a person with type O blood. All other blood types are incompatible with O recipients.

Blood type AB is the universal recipient; people with this blood type can theoretically accept an organ from any donor. However, people with this blood type can donate an organ only to another person with type AB blood.

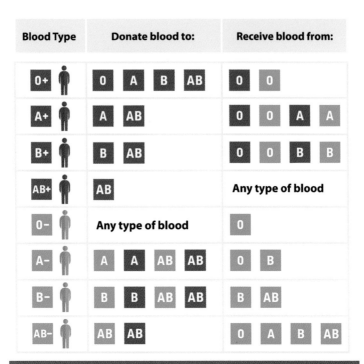

Blood Type	Donate blood to:	Receive blood from:
O+	O A B AB	O O
A+	A AB	O O A A
B+	B AB	O O B B
AB+	AB	Any type of blood
O–	Any type of blood	O
A–	A A AB AB	O B
B–	B B AB AB	B AB
AB–	AB AB	O A B AB

Once blood typing was established, transfusion and transplantation became much more successful.

Donors with blood type A can donate to recipients with type A or AB. Donors with blood type B can donate to recipients with type B or AB. Recipients with blood type A can only receive organs from a person with type A or O blood. Recipients with blood type B can receive only from a person with type B or O blood.

Once a match is found in terms of blood type, tissue-typing must be performed. All people have six basic antigens in their bodies, which they received from their parents. Antigens induce immune responses in the body, so in theory, if the antigens between donor and recipient don't match, the recipient's body may try to mount an immune response against the foreign organ. In the best-case scenario, the donor and recipient have six out of six matching antigens. However, transplants have been successfully performed on people with low antigen matches.

Finally, the donor and recipient both need to have a cross-match. This is a blood test that determines whether the recipient's body will attack the new organ. The test is performed at least twice before the transplant to ensure that the donor organ is likely to be a good match.

Aside from these tests, the medical team will evaluate the donor and recipient based on body size, length of time the recipient has been on the waiting list, and medical urgency. People who are likely to die soon without a transplant are often moved to the top of the waiting list, while less urgent cases are pushed down in the list. However, if the person at the top of the list doesn't seem like a good candidate for any reason, the transplant team will move on to the next likely match on the list. Teams work hard to ensure the most likely success for organ transplantation, especially since organs are in such short supply.

Body size isn't always a deal breaker. Sometimes it is because an adult organ may simply be too large to fit in the body of a child. This is the case with organs like the heart and lungs. But if it's a situation in which a partial transplant will be successful, then that's an option. For example, a portion of an adult liver can be transplanted into a child, and it will regrow into a full liver for the child.

All of these success factors for transplants have been determined after years of transplants, research, and scientific discovery. Organ transplantation has become much more successful as doctors and scientists have learned more about how the body is formed, works, and reacts to foreign tissues.

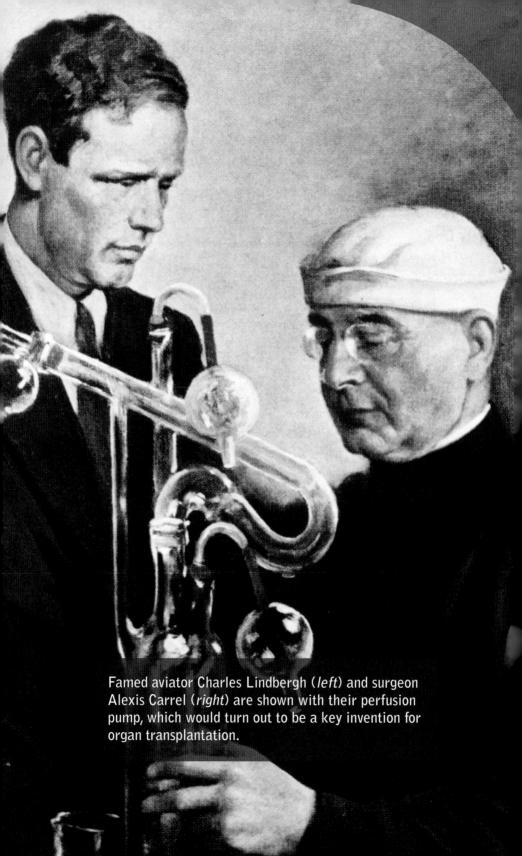

Famed aviator Charles Lindbergh (*left*) and surgeon Alexis Carrel (*right*) are shown with their perfusion pump, which would turn out to be a key invention for organ transplantation.

CHAPTER 3

The Major Players in Organ Transplants

Science almost never happens in a vacuum. Scientists are constantly learning about the research and discoveries of others in the field, and that informs their own research, work, and discoveries. It's like a team of people building a tower—some lay the foundation, many add to the structure, and ultimately a few people finish the top. Except that in scientific discovery, the top is really never finished. There's always something new to be discovered, new research to be done, and new applications to be explored.

This chapter covers some of the major contributors to the field of organ transplantation.

ALEXIS CARREL

Dr. Alexis Carrel was a French surgeon and biologist whose contributions to the surgical and transplant fields cannot be overstated. His first major contribution to the field came when he was a young surgeon, just twenty-one years old.

French president Marie-François-Sadi Carnot was stabbed and, ultimately, bled to death. The assassin's blade had severed Carnot's portal vein, and the surgeons who treated him were unable to successfully reattach it. Disturbed by this, Carrel used his knowledge of sewing, which he had learned when he took lessons from an embroideress, to develop a suturing technique for blood vessels known as triangulation.

This technique uses three stitches, each placed a third of the way around the circumference of the meeting of the two blood vessels. The three stitches are then retracted, which pulls the circular shape of the vessels into a triangle. The triangular shape is much easier to suture and minimizes potential damage to the walls of the blood vessels during suturing.

The triangulation technique, still used today, changed the face of vascular surgery. It even won Carrel the 1912 Nobel Prize in Physiology or Medicine. Organ transplant involves much suturing of blood vessels when organs are reconnected, so Carrel's innovation became incredibly useful in the field of organ transplantation as well.

Carrel's contributions to the field of organ transplantation didn't end there. In the 1930s, he worked with Charles Lindbergh to develop the perfusion pump, which was groundbreaking for organ transplantation.

The perfusion pump is what allows organs to remain viable outside the body during surgery. Outside the body, organs have a limited lifespan. The perfusion pump supplies organs with oxygenated blood or a synthetic substitute to keep them functioning as they await transplant into a recipient's body.

The Charles Lindbergh that Carrel collaborated with is the famed American aviator. Lindbergh was also an inventor. Carrel had reportedly developed the fluid to keep organs functioning but hadn't yet figured out how to mechanically apply it to organs. Lindbergh had great knowledge of mechanics and designed a three-chambered glass vessel that would hold the organ in place and allow Carrel's blood substitute to perfuse through it via air pressure, which is similar to how blood perfuses through the body in the natural biological process. (In case you're wondering what inspired Lindbergh to get involved with this invention, it was reportedly his sister-in-law's devastating diagnosis of severe heart disease that inspired him.)

The Carrel-Lindbergh team only made about twenty of the perfusion pumps, but they are considered to be the inspiration for important later medical devices such as the cardiopulmonary bypass pump, also known as a heart-lung machine. The process they used reportedly helped inform the process used to stop hearts during surgical procedures, such as heart transplants.

JOSEPH MURRAY

Together, doctors Joseph Murray and David Hume performed the first successful human kidney transplant. Kidney transplants had been attempted earlier but had been unsuccessful. Immunosuppressant drugs to effectively prevent organ rejection hadn't been established yet, which made successful transplants nearly impossible. But Murray and Hume performed the transplant on a pair of identical twins. Since the twins had identical DNA, there was very little risk of organ rejection.

Hume was a pioneer in kidney disease research and treatment, and he was part of the team that assisted Murray in the landmark five-and-a-half-hour operation at Peter Bent Brigham Hospital, in Boston. The recipient of the kidney, twin Richard Herrick, had been dying of chronic inflammation of the kidneys. He lived eight years after the transplant, dying at the age of thirty-one in 1963.

Murray was a young plastic surgeon when he performed the surgery—just thirty-five years old. He had attended Harvard Medical School and done his internship at Peter Bent Brigham. He joined the surgical staff at Peter Bent Brigham in 1951, after serving in the Medical Corps of the United States Army, just three years before performing the surgery.

Murray continued to work in the field of organ transplant after the surgery, studying immunosuppressant drugs and the mechanisms of organ rejection. He was part of the team that developed the immunosuppressant drug Imuran in 1957, which ultimately led to successful kidney transplants being performed between unrelated patients.

Much like Alexis Carrel before him, Joseph Murray was honored as a pioneer in the field of organ transplantation by receiving a Nobel Prize in Physiology or Medicine in 1990. Murray died at the age of ninety-three, after suffering a stroke on Thanksgiving Day, in 2012. Fittingly, he passed away in the very hospital where he had performed his groundbreaking surgery and inspired countless other doctors who later became leaders in the field of transplantation.

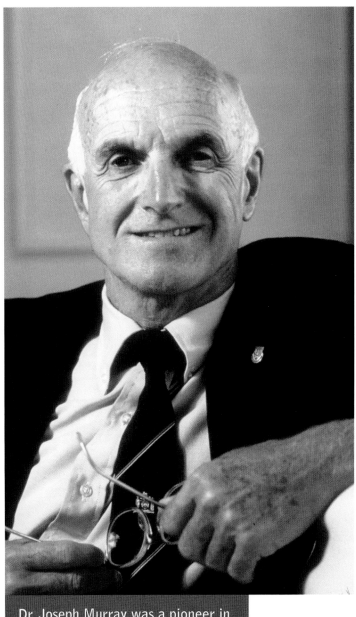

Dr. Joseph Murray was a pioneer in kidney transplantation.

JAMES HARDY

Dr. James Hardy was a surgeon at the University of Mississippi Medical Center, in Jackson, when he performed the world's first lung transplant in 1963. The surgery was not entirely successful. The patient, John Russell, lived for just eighteen days after the transplant. Still, Hardy is considered a pioneer in the field of organ transplant.

The surgery was somewhat controversial in large part because of the patient. John Russell was a convicted murderer serving a life sentence at the Mississippi State Penitentiary. He suffered from emphysema in both lungs, cancer in his left lung, kidney disease, and, at the time of the transplant, pneumonia that was not responding to antibiotic treatment. There is some question as to whether Russell received a reduced prison sentence for agreeing to allow the surgery to be performed, but Hardy denied that. It ended up being a moot point since Russell ultimately died eighteen days after the surgery.

During the surgery, Hardy and his team discovered that the cancer in Russell's left lung had spread, and thus the single-lung transplant would not save his life. However, it was hoped that he would have a better ability to breathe for his remaining days if the transplant were completed.

Indeed, the transplant did help Russell's breathing, and his body did not reject the lung, due to the use of immunosuppressant drugs, including the Imuran that pioneering doctor Joseph Murray had helped to develop. However, Russell's kidneys ultimately failed, and his death was reportedly due to cancer, infection, and kidney failure.

Still, the lung transplant was a step forward in organ transplantation since it does not appear that the transplanted lung caused Russell's death.

Hardy continued to work in transplantation, and the next year he performed the first heart transplant and the first xenotransplantation when he placed the heart of a chimpanzee into the body of dying patient Boyd Rush. The transplanted chimp heart beat for roughly sixty minutes before stopping. This surgery, too, was rather controversial because it's questionable whether Hardy informed Rush's family that a chimpanzee heart would be used. Hardy claimed that he had verbally discussed it with the family, but the hospital consent form did not state it in writing. So, it is questionable whether the one relative available at the time of the surgery, Rush's stepsister, knew that a chimpanzee heart would be used in her stepbrother.

Still, the fact that Hardy had managed to transplant a heart (from a chimpanzee, no less) and had gotten it to beat for an hour was an important step in organ transplant history.

THOMAS STARZL

Thomas Starzl is considered by many to be the father of modern organ transplantation. Starzl intended to become a priest, but his mother died of cancer when he was just twenty-one years old. That inspired Starzl to change his focus to medicine.

After earning a medical degree at Northwestern University Medical School, in Illinois, he trained in surgery

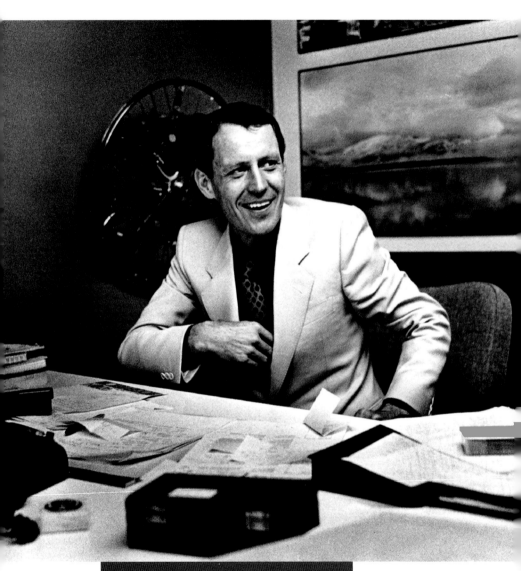

Dr. Thomas Starzl performed the first human liver transplant.

at Johns Hopkins Hospital, in Maryland, and at Jackson Memorial Hospital, in Florida. He became a surgeon and researcher in organ transplantation at the University of Colorado in 1962, and just a year later, he performed the first liver transplant.

Starzl's first attempt at a liver transplant, in 1963, was not successful. The patient was a child who died during surgery of uncontrolled bleeding. Other surgeons tried unsuccessfully to perform liver transplants over the next few years, but it wasn't until 1967 that a liver transplant was successful. That successful transplant was also performed by Dr. Starzl.

The recipient of the liver in the 1967 transplant was a nineteen-month-old child who lived for a year post-transplant. She ultimately died from the disease that had attacked her liver in the first place. But the liver transplant itself was successful. The disease is what ultimately claimed the patient's life.

Starzl was also instrumental in establishing the clinical use of the immunosuppressant cyclosporine in transplants in the 1980s. The use of cyclosporine led to much greater success in liver transplantation, which had suffered from an extremely low success rate prior to the use of drugs like cyclosporine.

In addition, Starzl helped develop numerous medical advances in organ preservation and transplantation. He also contributed to research on the role immunosuppressant drugs play in post-transplant infections and diseases.

Finally, in 1984, Starzl performed the first simultaneous heart and liver transplant. The patient was a six-year-old girl who had a rare disease that increased her cholesterol levels to ten times the normal level, resulting in liver disease and multiple heart attacks. The surgery was a success, and the patient lived four years with no complications. She began to have problems with the liver four years after the surgery. Ultimately, she required a second liver transplant in 1990, but it was due to hepatitis, not due to organ rejection. The second transplant was a success, but the patient died later that year due to rejection of the heart transplant Starzl had performed in 1984.

CHRISTIAAN BARNARD

Christiaan Barnard may be one of the most recognizable names in the world of organ transplantation. He is the cardiac surgeon who performed the first successful human-to-human heart transplant. The surgery took place in December 1967, at Groote Schuur Hospital, in Cape Town, South Africa.

Barnard did not actually begin his career as a cardiac surgeon. In his first years as a doctor, he worked in the gastrointestinal field, where he developed a lifesaving treatment for intestinal atresia, a birth defect affecting the small or large intestine.

In 1955, Barnard came to the United States to work more in the gastrointestinal field, but while there, he was introduced to Walt Lillehei, a pioneering surgeon in open-heart and cardiothoracic surgery. (In a bit of a coincidence, Walt Lillehei's younger brother, Richard, was actually part of the team that later performed the first successful kidney-pancreas transplant in 1966.) Barnard worked with Lillehei and then returned to South Africa, where he was named head of the Department of Experimental Surgery at Groote Schuur Hospital.

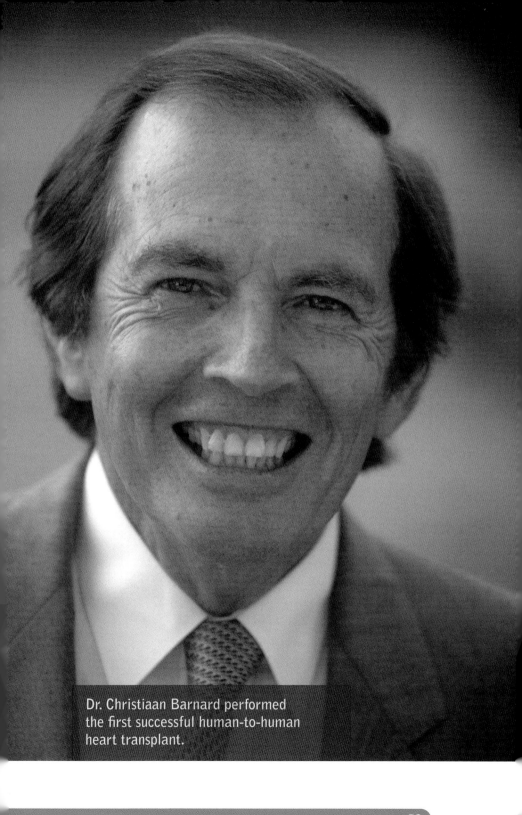

Dr. Christiaan Barnard performed the first successful human-to-human heart transplant.

The landmark 1967 surgery was somewhat successful. The patient lived for eighteen days and regained full consciousness before dying of pneumonia. The team concluded that the immunosuppressant drugs given to the patient post-transplant were a likely cause of the pneumonia that ultimately claimed his life.

Barnard performed a second heart transplant in 1968, and that patient lived for nineteen months before dying. Approximately one hundred other transplants were attempted by other surgeons that same year, with less-than-stellar results. Two-thirds of the patients died within the first three months after the transplant. As the years went on, though, there were successful transplants. In 1971, Barnard transplanted a heart into Cape Town resident Dirk van Zyl, who went on to live for twenty-three more years before dying of complications from a stroke. Interestingly, South Africa was extremely segregated at that time under apartheid laws. Van Zyl was a white man and thus eligible to receive treatment at Groote Schuur Hospital. However, his heart was from a mixed-race donor who would not have been eligible for treatment at the hospital.

Even though Barnard's success rate for transplants was inconsistent, his work in the field of heart transplantation was a major achievement in the organ transplant field. Nowadays, thousands of heart transplants are performed per year, and one-year survival rates are greater than 90 percent.

NORMAN SHUMWAY

While Christiaan Barnard performed the first successful heart transplant worldwide, the doctor behind the first successful heart transplant in the United States was heart surgeon Norman Shumway.

Like Barnard, Shumway studied under famed cardiothoracic surgeon Walt Lillehei. Shumway's first heart transplant was in 1968, just a year after Barnard's. Many cardiac surgeons stopped attempting heart transplants when they determined that success rates were low, but Shumway persisted. In the 1970s, he continued to study immunosuppressant drugs in an attempt to combat the possibility of rejection. He was a pioneer in the use of cyclosporine, the immunosuppressant that was approved for use in 1983 and drastically improved post-transplant outcomes. In 1981, Shumway partnered with Bruce Reitz to perform the world's first heart-lung transplant.

BRUCE REITZ

In 1981, cardiothoracic surgeon Bruce Reitz teamed with Shumway to perform the first heart-lung transplant, which took place at Stanford Hospital, in California. Reitz still teaches at Stanford University, and his current research interests include the study of organ rejection for heart and lung transplants and other topics related to immunosuppressant drugs and transplants.

Stanford University: At the Forefront of Transplant Research

The United States has stayed at the forefront of medical research in the field of organ transplantation. One institution that has contributed enormously to this field is Stanford University and its associated hospital, located in Palo Alto, California.

Cardiothoracic surgeon Bruce Reitz is part of why Stanford University and its associated hospital have remained at the forefront of transplant research and surgeries. Stanford is where the first adult heart transplant in the United States took place, when Norman Shumway performed the surgery in 1968. Reitz performed the first successful heart-lung transplant there in 1981. He recalled his early involvement in heart-lung transplants in an interview published in *Stanford Medicine*:

> [I]n 1969, when I was still a medical student, I asked about working in the research lab run by Dr. Norman Shumway, chief of the Division of Cardiothoracic Surgery and the father of heart transplantation. Eighteen months earlier, he and his team did the first successful adult heart transplant in the United States.

He said yes. After I finished my residency in cardiac surgery, I came back to the lab. I asked Dr. Shumway what needed to be done, and he said he'd like to see if we could make some progress in combining heart transplantation with complete bilateral lung transplantation. There were patients with congenital heart defects and patients with severe lung disease who currently could not be treated by transplantation. Mary Gohlke, whose heart had been damaged by her disease, was exactly that kind of patient. Nor did we have a way to transplant lungs then except as part of a heart-lung package.

Stanford is also known for its expertise in multi-organ transplants. They regularly perform heart, heart-lung, intestine, liver, lung, kidney, kidney-pancreas, and blood and bone marrow transplants. In addition to living donor transplants, they also perform partial organ transplants and transplants from cadavers.

EDWARD DONNALL THOMAS

Edward Donnall Thomas shared the 1990 Nobel Prize in Physiology or Medicine with Joseph Murray (the surgeon who performed the first successful kidney transplant) for his work in bone marrow transplantation. While leading a team at the Fred Hutchinson Cancer Research Center at the University of Washington, in Seattle, Thomas determined that transplanted bone marrow stem cells could repopulate blood cells in the bone marrow of a recipient. The team's work also helped lower the number of patients suffering from graft-versus-host disease, which is essentially rejection of the transplanted marrow cells.

Bone marrow transplantation was an important step in treating leukemia, a cancer of the blood cells.

JOEL D. COOPER

Thoracic surgeon Joel D. Cooper is notable for having performed both the first successful single-lung transplant and the first successful double-lung transplant.

The single-lung transplant took place in November 1983, at Toronto General Hospital, in Ontario, Canada, on a man suffering from pulmonary fibrosis. Three years later, at the same hospital, Cooper performed the first successful double-lung transplant on a woman suffering from emphysema. The woman went on to live for nearly fifteen years post-transplant before dying of an unrelated brain aneurysm.

He currently heads the thoracic surgery department at the University of Pennsylvania, in Philadelphia, where he continues his work in the field of lung transplants and related surgeries.

CHRISTOPH BROELSCH

German surgeon Christoph Broelsch was the first surgeon to successfully transplant a segment of a liver. The surgery was performed in January 1988, and the four-month old patient is still alive and living in the United States.

VAUGHN A. STARNES

Cardiothoracic surgeon Vaughn A. Starnes gained recent fame in 2017 when late-night talk show host Jimmy Kimmel shared a story about how Starnes and his team at Children's Hospital of Los Angeles performed lifesaving heart surgery on Kimmel's infant son, who was born with holes in his heart and a blocked pulmonary valve.

However, earlier in his career, Starnes was notable for performing the first transplant of a lung lobe donated from a living donor in 1990. The donor was a mother, and the recipient was her preteen daughter.

In 1993, Starnes also performed the first double-lobe transplant from a live donor. In that case, a child with cystic fibrosis received a transplant of two lung lobes—one from each of the child's parents.

SATORU TODO, ANDREAS G. TZAKIS, and JOHN FUNG

In 1992, led by pioneering transplant surgeon Thomas Starzl, the team of doctors Satoru Todo, Andreas G. Tzakis, and John Fung performed the world's first successful baboon-to-human liver transplant at University of Pittsburgh Hospital, in Pennsylvania. Xenograft transplants had to that point been wholly unsuccessful, so the fact that the patient, who had been dying of hepatitis B, ultimately lived for two months and regained consciousness was a major step forward in the research.

The last animal-to-human transplant before the 1992 experimental surgery took place in 1984, when surgeons at Loma Linda Medical Center, in California, transplanted a baboon heart into an infant, who lived only twenty days. That infant, known as "Baby Fae," had received the immunosuppressant cyclosporine, which is typically very effective for human-to-human transplants. It had, however, not worked in the case of Baby Fae, so the team in 1992 decided to select four other antirejection drugs they felt would work better in a xenograft transplant.

The surgery was performed in part because hepatitis B tends to attack newly transplanted livers in the same way it attacks the diseased liver. The team hoped that the baboon liver would not be susceptible to hepatitis B. Indeed, the liver did not appear to suffer ill effects from hepatitis B—the recipient developed an infection that grew quickly due to an overdose of antirejection drugs.

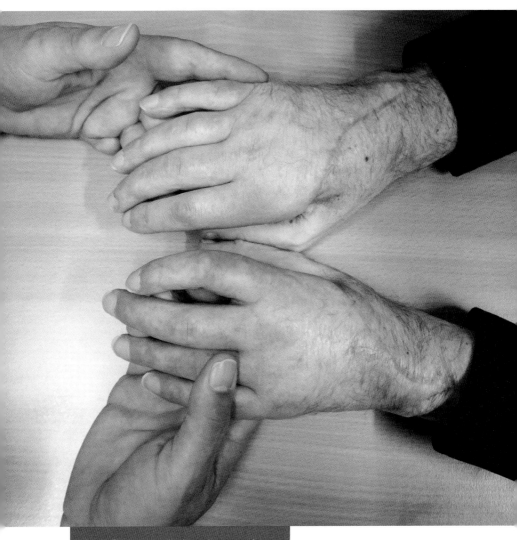

The first double hand transplant done in the United Kingdom is shown on the right.

A second human-to-baboon transplant was performed in 1993, but that recipient never regained consciousness and died less than a month later from an infection.

EARL OWEN and JEAN-MICHEL DUBERNARD

In 1998, microsurgeon Earl Owen from Australia and doctor Jean-Michel Dubernard from France performed the first successful hand transplant. The success of the surgery was short-lived because the recipient, a man from New Zealand, did not follow the appropriate post-transplant drug therapy and physiotherapy. He wasn't pleased with the functioning of the hand and requested that the team remove it in 2001, after an episode of rejection.

However, the surgery was technically a success, and it paved the way for future successful hand transplants. Hand transplants are notoriously difficult and time-consuming because the team must reconnect bones, tendons, arteries, nerves, veins, and skin. This process takes about eight to twelve hours, compared to the six to eight hours a typical heart transplant takes.

BERNARD DEVAUCHELLE

Face transplants are one of the newest types of transplants to be performed. French maxillofacial surgeon Bernard Devauchelle performed the first successful partial face transplant in 2005, at Amiens University Hospital in France. On his team, Devauchelle also worked with Jean-Michel Dubernard, who was on the team of the first successful hand transplant.

The recipient of the partial face transplant was a French woman who had been mauled by her dog in 2005. The team grafted a triangle of facial tissue from a brain-dead donor onto her nose, chin, and mouth. The surgery was a success, but it was very difficult. The recipient experienced issues with rejection. Unfortunately, due to the strong immunosuppressant drugs she had to take to prevent rejection of the tissue, she became more susceptible to illness and ultimately battled two types of cancer. She died eleven years after the transplant, from what was reported as a "long illness."

Without the contributions of these important doctors and researchers, organ transplantation would not be as evolved and successful as it is today. Next, we will look at how organ transplantation became a reality, and we will learn about the different types of transplants that exist today.

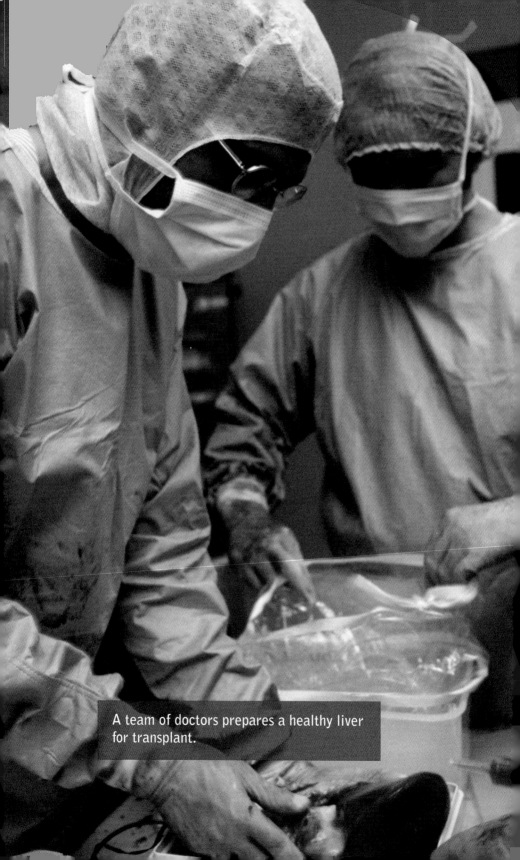

A team of doctors prepares a healthy liver for transplant.

CHAPTER 4

The Discovery of Organ Transplants

O nce the building blocks were in place and scientists began to understand how each organ in the body functions, how it's formed, and how it relies on or contributes to the functioning of other organs in the body, transplantation became a viable reality. Because there are so many different types of transplants and different organs, the first successful transplant didn't mean that transplantation was a reality for all organs. Rather, the major discovery of transplant science happened in a series of systematic steps.

DIFFERENT TYPES of TRANSPLANTS

There isn't just one type of organ transplant that is performed during an organ transplantation. Rather, there are several types.

Autograft

When the donor and recipient are the same person for a tissue transplant, it's known as an autograft. This type of transplant is highly desirable because the chance for rejection is nonexistent—the body recognizes the tissue as its own. In a similar type of transplant, called an isograft, the donor tissue comes from the recipient's identical twin. The chance for rejection in this type is very minimal.

Autografts are often done for skin grafts. The skin is technically an organ (the body's largest organ, in fact), and it regenerates all the time. When a person is injured in some way or skin cells die as part of the normal process of life, new skin cells generate. So, when a person needs a skin graft on a substantial patch of skin, due to a burn, a severe skin infection, removal of patches of skin cancer, or a significant wound, it's a common practice to take skin from another part of the body and graft it over the affected area.

The first successful skin graft surgery was performed in 1823, though there are reports of it being done as early as the first century in India. Needless to say, the procedure has been around for a long time, and it is done often and with great success.

Skin is not the only tissue that can be transplanted by autograft. Veins can be transplanted for coronary artery bypass grafting, a procedure done when the coronary artery is blocked.

Sometimes the autograft isn't immediate. Blood and stem cells can be banked, or stored, in anticipation of future use. Parents are starting to bank stem cell–rich umbilical cord blood as a sort of insurance that if their child or anyone else in the family needs a stem-cell transplant in the future, the cells will be available.

Regular blood can be banked as well. If a person is anticipating a surgery that may require a blood transfusion, he or she can bank the blood ahead of time rather than relying on donor blood from another person.

A rare surgery called a rotationplasty also uses autografting. In that surgery, a joint is used to replace another joint that is being removed due to partial limb amputation. For example, the ankle joint can be moved to take the place of a knee joint.

Allograft

Another common type of graft or transplant is the allograft, also sometimes called an allotransplant. This procedure involves transplanting tissue or an organ between two different people. When someone receives a donor kidney, for example, it's an allotransplant. (The exception is if the donor is an identical twin. Then, as mentioned, it's called an isograft.)

Allotransplants account for most transplants. Autografts are done whenever possible, but there are many cases in which an autograft simply isn't possible. A person cannot donate a heart or lung to themselves, for example!

Allotransplants have a reasonably high success rate now, but there is always the risk of organ rejection since the recipient's body sees the transplanted tissue or organ as foreign and will mount an immune response against it.

Xenograft

Xenografts, also called xenotransplants, are tissue or organ transplants between species. Humans obviously belong to the same species, so any human-to-human transplant is an allotransplant or autograft. But certain transplants do involve cross-species transplantation.

One common example is using a pig's heart valve in place of a human heart valve. This surgery generally has a high success rate, and the benefit to it is that the recipient does not have to be on anticoagulants, or blood thinners. The downside is that a pig valve typically lasts only ten to twenty years, so the recipient will likely need a replacement valve in a decade or two.

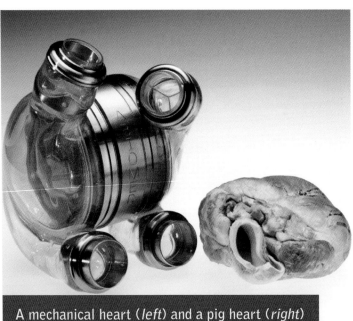

A mechanical heart (*left*) and a pig heart (*right*) are possible solutions for people waiting for heart transplants.

An alternative to pig valves is using mechanical valves as a replacement. These valves are long-lasting, but they usually require the recipient to be on anticoagulants for the rest of his or her life. Anticoagulants have some significant side effects, so lifetime dependence on them isn't desirable. Also, with mechanical valves, the risk for clotting is much greater, which is why anticoagulants are needed. Clots can be deadly if they dislodge and move through the bloodstream to the heart, lungs, or brain.

Xenotransplants are not very common because the success rate is very small. The chance of rejection is very high. There's also a risk of an animal-carried disease being transferred to the human recipient. Currently, most research on xenotransplants is being done with human-to-animal transplants—that is, using donor organs from deceased humans and transplanting them into animals to try to study how xenotransplantation might be possible in the future. In this way, human patients are not harmed. (The donor organs are ones that are not compatible with a human currently waiting for a transplant—either the organ is not suitable for transplant or there's no waiting match.)

Domino Transplant

The phrase "domino transplant" refers to a sort of domino effect with transplant. Some transplants have higher success rates when multiple organs are transplanted at once. For example, pancreas transplants usually also involve the kidneys, and for patients needing a double-lung transplant, it's often more successful to do a heart-and-double-lung transplant.

In these cases, if one of the recipient's organs involved in the transplant is healthy, it will be removed and donated to another recipient. For example, people with cystic fibrosis often require double-lung transplants, but their hearts are often healthy. Because the heart-lung transplant is easier and more successful than just a double-lung transplant, the heart and lungs will come from one donor and be placed into the recipient with cystic fibrosis. The healthy heart from the person with cystic fibrosis will then be transplanted into another recipient. It's an unusual but mutually beneficial situation for the living donor and both recipients!

Sometimes domino transplants are also done when a person has an organ that will not last for his or her lifetime but would last for a recipient's lifetime. For example, if a young person has a disease that very slowly destroys the liver, he or she will need a liver transplant. If the transplant is done early enough that the diseased liver is still relatively healthy, then that diseased liver can be donated to an older person whose life will likely end for other reasons long before the slow-moving disease destroys the liver.

Although it seems odd to think about transplanting a diseased organ, in some cases it will buy an older recipient a little more time. This was the case when the Mayo Clinic, in Rochester, Minnesota, performed a domino transplant with a liver in 2003. The donor with the diseased liver was only forty-three, and the recipient was sixty-four and had a different liver disease that would have claimed his life much more quickly. Receiving the liver with the slow-moving disease is thought to have bought him twenty to thirty more years. According to the United Network for Organ Sharing (UNOS), given that sixteen people in the United States die each day while waiting for transplants, the domino transplant was a viable solution.

ABO-Incompatible Transplant

The problem with incompatible organs is how the immune system responds to the transplant. A heart from an adult with type A blood cannot be transplanted into an adult recipient with type B blood, for example. The recipient's immune system will reject the organ.

The exception to this rule is young children—the younger the better, but sometimes children up to two years old can be good candidates for what's called an ABO-incompatible transplant. Young children have not yet developed strong immune systems, so their bodies are less likely to reject an incompatible organ. Specifically, very young children have low levels of T-cell-independent antigens and do not have isohemagglutinins, which are substances that agglutinate red blood cells. When the ratio of isohemagglutinin in a child's blood is 1:4 or less, that child may be allowed to receive an ABO-incompatible transplant. However, if there is an ABO match for the donor organ, that recipient will receive the organ instead of the ABO-incompatible recipient. Once again, it's a matter of the donor organ going to the recipient who is most likely to be a good match with the lowest chance of organ rejection.

Sometimes, ABO-incompatible transplants can work in adults, but typically not with major organs like the heart. Success is much better in kidney transplants. However, ABO-incompatible transplants are not a preferred choice. If a matching organ is available, it's a much better option.

Donor Chains

Domino transplants also occur in what are called donor chains. These can work in the case of living transplants, such as kidney transplants. The goal is to increase the availability of organs for transplantation.

Some people awaiting transplants have potential donors, but those donors don't end up being a match for them. In a coordinated effort, the willing donor can instead donate the organ to someone else on the transplant list, with the understanding that his or her relative on the transplant list will receive a donation from an unknown donor.

It's a complicated, coordinated effort that was pioneered by well-known medical institutions Johns Hopkins Medical Center, in Baltimore, Maryland, and Northwestern Memorial Hospital, in Chicago, Illinois. In 2011 and 2012, in a coordinated four-month effort, sixty donors and recipients participated in the longest donor chain thus far. A total of thirty patients received a kidney from a living donor.

It started with a man in California who agreed to donate a kidney to a stranger. The recipient was a man in New York. That recipient's niece, who had wanted to donate her kidney to him but was not a match, then donated her kidney to a young woman in Wisconsin. The chain progressed, with family members of recipients each donating a kidney to a stranger, until the final patient, a diabetic man in Chicago, received his kidney.

In total, the donor chain took four months, thirty donors and thirty recipients, countless doctors and other medical professionals, the involvement of eleven states and seventeen hospitals, and a lot of coast-to-coast flights with kidneys carefully packed for transport. But many lives were improved, and available organs were maximized. While domino transplants may not be the most efficient way to handle the issue of a shortage of organs for transplantation, it has enabled many people to live long, healthy lives.

TRANSPLANT FIRSTS

Organ transplantation wasn't discovered all at once.
Rather, doctors successfully performed certain transplants
or procedures, which led to future success with other
transplantation developments. It's a series of building blocks
that have led to where the field is today.

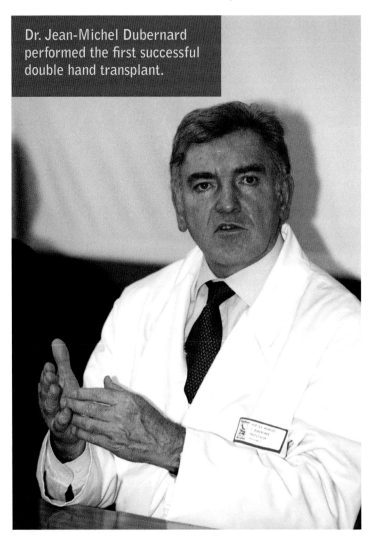

Dr. Jean-Michel Dubernard
performed the first successful
double hand transplant.

Technically, the first transplant was a skin graft performed in 1823 by Dr. Carl Bunger. It was an autograft. Dr. Bunger grafted flesh from a patient's inner thigh onto the patient's nose, which had been destroyed by the disease syphilis. Because the donor and recipient were the same person, and it was a relatively small section of skin, the graft was a success.

Next, Dr. Theodor Kocher transplanted thyroid tissue in 1883. Then, just after the turn of the twentieth century, Dr. Alexis Carrel of France began to perform autografts of veins and arteries, pioneering a vascular-suturing technique that is still used today.

Shortly thereafter, in 1905, Dr. Eduard Zirm performed the first successful corneal transplant, using donor corneas from a boy whose eyes had been damaged when iron became lodged in both eyes. The boy's eyes had to be removed, and Zirm used the corneas for another patient whose corneas had been destroyed while working with a type of caustic lime (the mineral, not the fruit). The transplant was successful in one of two eyes.

There were several decades of failed transplant attempts, until Dr. Richard Lawler performed a successful kidney transplant in 1950. However, that transplant was not successful long-term—it failed ten months later. Four years later, though, Dr. Joseph Murray did successfully perform a kidney transplant. It was an isograft, in which a kidney was taken from one brother and transplanted into his identical twin, drastically reducing the chances of rejection.

In the early 1960s, immunosuppressive drugs began to be used, and consequently, a cadaver-to-living-human kidney transplant performed by the same Dr. Joseph Murray was successful in 1962. The following year, Dr. James Hardy performed the first technically successful lung transplant, though the recipient ended up living only eighteen days, so it wasn't a long-term success.

That failure didn't stop Hardy from trying, though. The very next year, he attempted the first heart transplant (and a xenotransplant, at that!) when he transplanted a chimpanzee heart into a human. The heart did beat for an hour once transplanted, but then it stopped.

Riding on the success of kidney transplants performed by Dr. Joseph Murray, doctors Richard Lillehei and William Kelly performed the first successful kidney-pancreas transplant in 1966. This surgery is still widely done because when a pancreas transplant is needed, the patient's kidneys are often also damaged or diseased. Interestingly, the first successful isolated pancreas transplant didn't happen until 1968 (again by Dr. Lillehei). So, the multi-organ transplant actually happened before the single-organ transplant, in this case.

In 1967, Dr. Thomas Starzl performed the first successful liver transplant, and that same year, Dr. Christiaan Barnard of South Africa performed the first successful heart transplant. In 1968, Dr. Norman Shumway performed the first successful heart transplant in the United States.

That same year, the first successful bone marrow transplant was performed by Dr. E. Donnall Thomas. Marrow transplants are a standard treatment now for leukemia and other blood diseases, and it is a promising part of stem-cell research.

In 1981, another multi-organ transplant milestone was reached when doctors Bruce Reitz and Norman Shumway

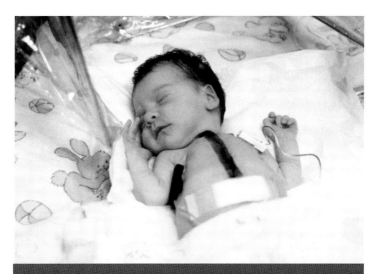

Baby Fae was the first infant to undergo a heart transplant from a baboon. She died twenty-one days after the surgery.

performed the first successful heart-lung transplant. Once again, the multi-organ transplant was successfully performed before a single-organ transplant in the case of the lungs. The first successful single-lung transplant was performed two years later, in 1983, by Dr. Joel Cooper. Three years later, he performed the first double-lung transplant.

In 1984, successful xenotransplantation became a reality when Baby Fae, as she was nicknamed, received a baboon heart transplant. She lived for one month with the baboon heart, making it a successful transplant even though the success wasn't long term. The same thing happened with a baboon-to-human liver transplant attempted in 1992, but in that case, the recipient lived two months post-transplant.

Another milestone was reached in 1989, when Dr. Christoph Broelsch performed the first successful transplant of a segment of a liver. Given that liver cells can regenerate, it's possible to successfully transplant only a portion of the organ. The same holds true for lungs—there are cases in which only a single lobe of a lung can be transplanted successfully. The first successful transplant of this type was performed by Dr. Vaughn Starnes in 1990.

In 1998, the first successful hand transplant was performed by doctors Earl Owen and Jean-Michel Dubernard. The transplant was incredibly complicated because of the number of nerves, tendons, and blood vessels involved in the hand. The transplant took place in France, with the first successful United States hand transplant taking place in 2001.

In 2005, the first successful partial face transplant became a reality, with Dr. Jean-Michel Dubernard again part of the team. In 2010, a team of thirty doctors in Spain performed the first full-face transplant.

As you can see, the discoveries in organ transplantation have been numerous and spread out over many decades, with each milestone reached contributing to the next discovery.

The IMPORTANCE of IMMUNOSUPPRESSANT DRUGS

Immunosuppressant drugs have multiple uses. They aren't only used to prevent organ rejection. But preventing organ rejection is one major use for them, and the success rates of organ transplants have improved drastically since immunosuppressants were introduced.

There are two types of immunosuppressants: induction drugs and maintenance drugs. Induction drugs are administered right at the time of the transplant. Maintenance drugs are a long-term solution to try to prevent organ rejection. The majority of organ recipients will be on maintenance immunosuppressants for the rest of their lives. The only exception is people who received an organ from an identical twin; they may or may not have to take long-term immunosuppressants.

Even missing one daily dose of an immunosuppressant increases the recipient's risk of rejecting the organ. The immune system is *that* powerful. If the immunosuppressant regimen isn't followed as closely as possible, the chance for rejection increases.

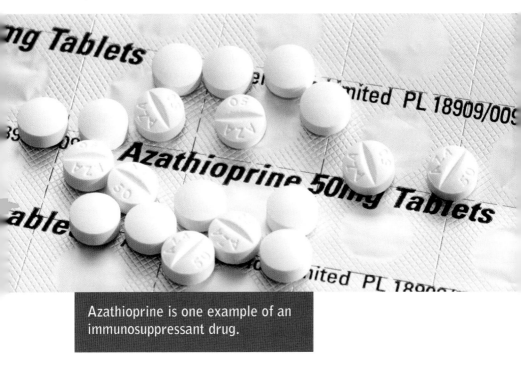

Azathioprine is one example of an immunosuppressant drug.

Even with immunosuppressants, organ rejection can still occur. It's far less likely, but it can still happen.

Immunosuppressants are a bit of a necessary evil as far as transplant is concerned. Without them, organ rejection is almost certain. But with them, a person's immune system is compromised, and he or she becomes more vulnerable to infection and illness. This is because an immunosuppressant does exactly what it sounds like: it suppresses the immune system. In addition to fighting against donor organs, the immune system fights against all foreign invaders, such as viruses and bacteria. So, people on immunosuppressants must take extra precautions not to unnecessarily expose themselves to illness.

In the early days of transplants, doctors and scientists began to learn about organ rejection and experiment with methods for preventing it. They tried total body radiation, but that was a failure—all of the patients died. This is not surprising, given the fact that radiation has very strong negative effects on the body.

Doctors also tried steroids alone, but that didn't work either. Steroids are designed to reduce inflammation, and inflammation activates white blood cells to fight against foreign invaders. So, the theory is good, but it turns out that steroids alone are not enough to prevent organ rejection, as doctors soon learned. Steroids are still sometimes used to prevent organ rejection, but now they are used in combination with other immunosuppressive drugs.

In the early 1960s, Purinethol (mercaptopurine) was introduced as an immunosuppressant and chemotherapy drug. Imuran, another immunosuppressant that is also used to treat conditions that have chronic inflammation as a symptom, was introduced around the same time. Both began to be used as the standard treatment to try to prevent organ rejection.

During this time, scientists developed methods to closely match donor tissue to recipients, which helped improve transplant outcomes. Armed with this new knowledge, doctors began to routinely prescribe a combination of Imuran and steroids to prevent organ rejection. When combined with a good tissue match between donor and recipient, this seemed to work fairly well.

Later in the 1960s, targeted immunotherapy began. Scientists began to develop monoclonal and polyclonal antibodies to target specific immunoregulatory sites. These antibodies can bind to specific antigens and, in theory, prevent them from stimulating an immune response.

In 1983, the release of Cyclosporine was a huge step toward greater success with organ transplants. Cyclosporine (and similar drugs developed after it) are inhibitors. In the case of Cyclosporine, the drug inhibits a specific activity of a calcineurin that then decreases the function of white blood cells. Doctors began using Cyclosporine along with Imuran and steroids to provide a combined approach to immunosuppression. In doing so, they found greatly improved outcomes for organ transplant recipients.

Currently, immunosuppressants are used in two phases: induction and maintenance. The induction phase starts when the transplant takes place and immediately after. Maintenance then continues for the rest of the person's life.

Calcineurin inhibitors, such as Cyclosporine and the more recent Tacrolimus, are still widely used in transplants as primary immunosuppressants. Steroids are still widely

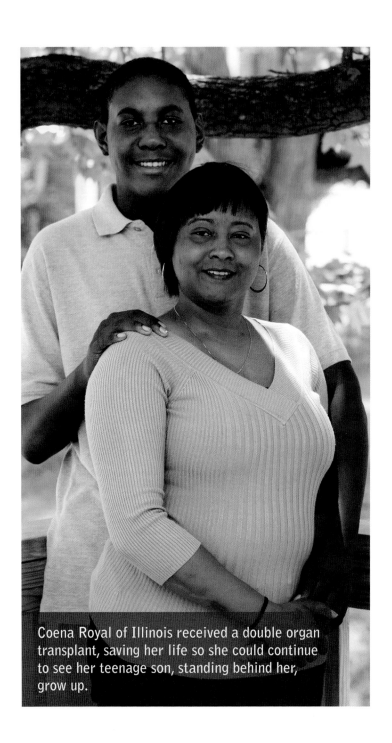

Coena Royal of Illinois received a double organ transplant, saving her life so she could continue to see her teenage son, standing behind her, grow up.

used as well to reduce inflammation and lower the likelihood of an immune response.

Imuran has been largely replaced by CellCept or similar drugs that act as adjuvant agents. Adjuvant agents modify the effects of other drugs being used. In the case of organ transplantation, adjuvant agents like CellCept help doctors decrease the toxicity of the other immunosuppressive drugs the patient is on.

The induction phase also often includes the use of monoclonal or polyclonal antibodies to prevent early acute rejection of the organ. However, these antibodies can have significant side effects, so sometimes doctors will choose instead to use aggressive doses of maintenance drugs in the induction phase to prevent rejection.

Without the advances in immunosuppressive drugs, there is little chance that organ transplantation would be anywhere near as successful as it is today. The human immune system is so good at detecting foreign invaders and fighting them that immunosuppression is the only way to override that.

However, we never know what the future might hold in the field of organ transplantation.

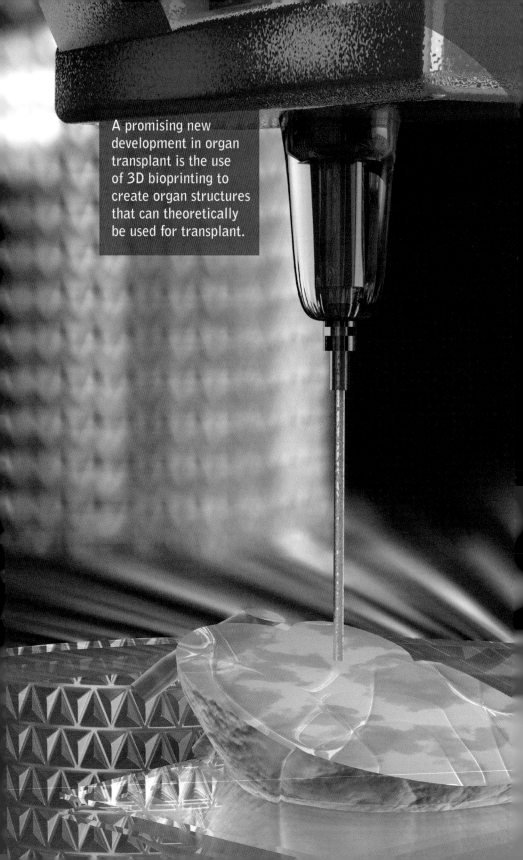

A promising new development in organ transplant is the use of 3D bioprinting to create organ structures that can theoretically be used for transplant.

CHAPTER 5

Organ Transplants Today

O rgan transplantation is still a very relevant field today. Every day, lives are saved or improved by transplants. The future looks bright, with new technologies holding promise for further developments and successes in the field.

SOME FACTS ABOUT TRANSPLANTS TODAY

The statistics about transplants change practically by the minute, given that an estimated eighty-one organ transplants take place each day in the United States. However, the United Network for Organ Sharing (UNOS) keeps meticulous records that are updated nearly daily.

UNOS Data

According to UNOS, from 1988 through early 2018, there have been more than 724,000 transplants in the United States. Kidney transplants account for nearly 59 percent of those

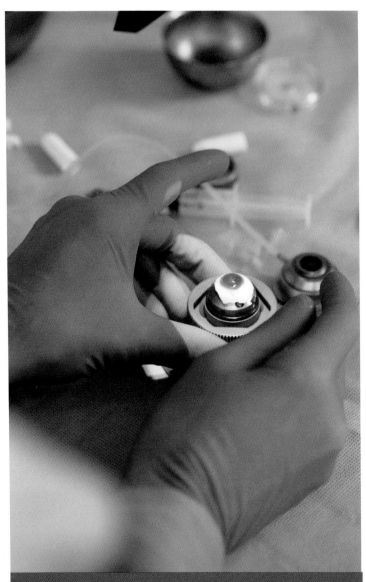

In the world of transplants, corneal transplants are relatively low-risk and common.

transplants, with more than 426,000 performed. The second most frequent transplant is of the liver; more than 156,000 have been transplanted in the United States since 1988.

Heart transplants are third most common, with nearly 70,000 performed since 1988. Lungs follow, with more than 36,000 lung transplants performed. Combination heart-lung transplants since 1988 number more than 1,200, and combination kidney-pancreas transplants number nearly 23,000. Pancreas-only transplants are much lower, at more than 8,000 performed since 1988.

Intestinal transplants come in at nearly 3,000 performed in the last thirty years. The remaining types of transplants, including head and neck, scalp, uterus, limb, and penis transplants, number ten or fewer in the past thirty years.

Perhaps the number of kidney transplants is so large because that is also the transplant with the most people on the waiting list, according to current UNOS data. As of early 2018, there were more than 95,000 people in the United States waiting for kidneys, more than 13,000 waiting for livers, nearly 4,000 waiting for hearts, more than 1,300 waiting for lungs, and nearly 900 waiting for pancreases. For combined transplants, there were more than 1,600 waiting for a kidney-pancreas transplant and more than 40 waiting for a heart-lung transplant as of early 2018.

Of those people waiting for transplants, more than 67 percent are age fifty or older. Adults who are thirty-five to forty-nine years old account for nearly 23 percent of the waiting list. The remaining 10 percent of people on the waiting list are under the age of thirty-five, with more than 8 of that 10 percent being young adults who are eighteen to thirty-four years old.

According to UNOS, an average of twenty people on the transplant waiting lists die each day while waiting for organs to become available. The lists keep growing because roughly every ten minutes, another person is added to the national transplant waiting list. As of early 2018, UNOS estimated that more than 115,000 people in the United States needed a lifesaving organ transplant, and the waiting list had nearly 75,000 active candidates. There is a definite imbalance between supply and demand—there are always more waiting candidates than there are donors. However, one donor can potentially save eight lives, if all of the donor's vital organs are usable and there is a match for a waiting recipient, which is not always the case. For example, in January 2018, UNOS recorded 2,853 transplants from 1,410 donors, meaning each donor donated, on average, two organs. Still, that's many lives saved that wouldn't otherwise have been. Up to seventy-five lives can be enhanced by non-lifesaving tissue donation. In fact, more than one million tissue transplants take place each year in the United States.

UNOS has also been tracking donations by donor type for the past several years. From 2013 through 2017, the majority of donors have been deceased. In 2017, for example, just over 6,100 transplants were from living donors, whereas more than 28,000 were from deceased donors. Living donors can provide a kidney or portions of the liver, lung, pancreas, or intestine.

UNOS also keeps track of where transplant centers are located and where organ-procurement organizations are located. Many states don't have organ-procurement organizations, but most have at least one organ transplant center. However, the distribution of organ transplant centers isn't always predictable. California, a very large and heavily populated state, has twenty-two organ transplant centers. Similarly, Texas has twenty-five. However, the largest state in the United States, Alaska, has none. Yet Massachusetts, a relatively small state, has nine. This seemingly random distribution may have something to do with the medical institutions in particular states. Massachusetts is home to a number of highly acclaimed universities and medical centers, so it stands to reason that those institutions might be at the forefront of this developing field. Indeed, looking at a map of transplant centers in Massachusetts reveals that all but two are clustered in or close to Boston, home to numerous universities and medical centers. Alaska, on the other hand, has hospitals and universities but none particularly known for being at the cutting edge of medical research.

The Truth About Transplants

Skeptics of organ transplantation have sometimes circulated theories about the practice, many of which are false. Some skeptics speculate that if a critically injured patient comes into a hospital, the trauma team sees them as a potential organ donor and does not make every effort to save the patient's life. This is not true. The number one priority of all hospitals is saving lives. If, however, a critically injured patient's life cannot be saved, then doctors who are not involved in organ and tissue donation are brought in to declare the patient brain dead. Only at that point can the medical team begin officially discussing donation options. But sometimes the patient's family, knowing their loved one is unlikely to live, will make the patient's wishes known earlier.

There is also no way to jump ahead on the transplant list. Wealth or celebrity status does not earn anyone a higher place on the list. In the 1990s, well-known actor Larry Hagman received a liver transplant because his liver had been badly damaged by severe cirrhosis resulting from alcoholism. At the time, some people felt he should not have been given a transplant because his liver failure was a result of alcohol abuse and an unhealthy lifestyle—some even wondered if his fame and wealth had allowed him to get it. The reality, though, is that Hagman was on the list and simply happened to be a match for a donor liver. The transplant gave Hagman an additional seventeen years of life, but he eventually succumbed to throat cancer, which doctors attributed to the immunosuppressant drugs he had to take after the transplant as well as the fact that he continued to drink alcohol even after the transplant. Not surprisingly, recipients of liver transplants are strongly advised not to drink alcohol, but, like Hagman, some whose livers were damaged due to alcohol abuse relapse post-transplant and begin drinking again.

Technically, it is against federal law to sell organs or tissues. So, it is highly unlikely that any licensed transplant center would even consider wealth as a factor in organ transplantation. Otherwise, the center might be accused of selling organs.

There are very few barriers to becoming an organ donor. There is no cost to the donor or donor's family, and in some states, even people under the age of eighteen can register as an organ donor. (However, if a person under eighteen is actually in a position to donate an organ, whether as a living donor or due to death, the person's legal guardian must consent to the donation.)

Anyone of any age, ethnicity, or medical history can, in theory, be a donor. Even noncitizens of the United States (nonresident aliens, for immigration purposes) can donate or receive organs. However, a few illnesses will prevent someone from being a donor, such as HIV, a systemic infection, or active cancer.

The FUTURE of ORGAN TRANSPLANTS

Technology in general is changing quickly, and that is also true in the field of organ transplantation. In the roughly fifty years since the first successful organ transplants, the technology has advanced greatly, and it shows no signs of slowing. There are some exciting developments on the horizon.

Growing Organs from Stem Cells

Stem cells show incredible promise for the field of medicine in general because they're so versatile. They are undifferentiated cells that can be edited to perform nearly any specific cell function. Scientists are even experimenting with growing organs for transplant out of a patient's own stem cells. This would allow patients to receive transplants with no risk of rejecting the organ.

In 2008, a Colombian woman, Claudia Castillo, received a transplant of a windpipe grown from her own stem cells.

Potential Application of Human Stem Cells

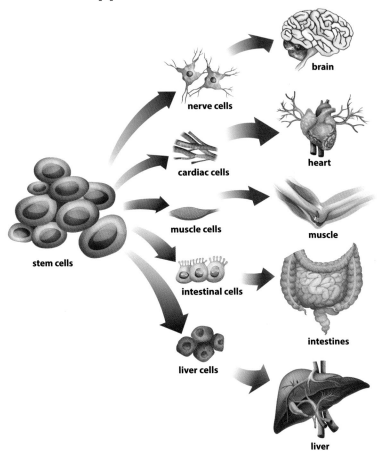

While scientists still experiment with stem-cell technology, the potential applications for organ transplantation are many.

A donor windpipe was stripped of cells, and Castillo's stem cells were used to grow an entirely new windpipe around the structure of the donor windpipe. While the transplant was only a temporary success (and the doctor who performed it has been under investigation for misconduct), it's an interesting look at a possible future technology.

Printing 3D Organs

A recent technological development is 3D printers, which do exactly what the name suggests: they print three-dimensional objects. A subset of this technology is 3D

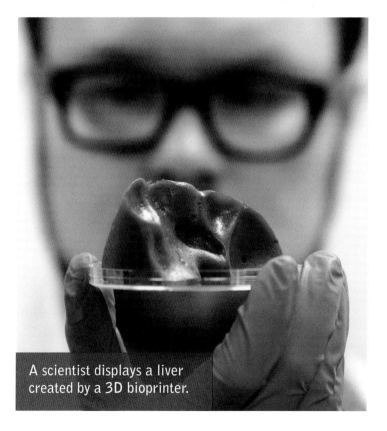

A scientist displays a liver created by a 3D bioprinter.

The Ethics of Disability and Transplants

While organ recipients are decided based on factors such as age, body size, blood type, and urgency of need, and factors like money and fame cannot determine when someone will receive a transplant, there is a situation that can unfairly influence whether one is on the transplant list: disability. People with physical and intellectual disabilities are sometimes denied a place on the transplant list even though there are federal laws in place to prevent that from happening. At the federal level, the Americans with Disabilities Act (ADA) prevents public facilities and state-run programs, such as many hospitals and transplant centers, from discriminating against people with disabilities. The federal Rehabilitation Act prohibits federally funded programs—one of which is the United Network for Organ Sharing—from discriminating against people with disabilities.

In fact, according to a survey done in 2004, 48 percent of people with an intellectual or developmental disability who asked to be referred to an organ transplant specialist ended up getting a referral. Of that 48 percent, 33 percent got the referral, but they were never actually evaluated by the organ transplant specialist.

How does this happen, despite federal protections? Sometimes medical professionals will turn down a disabled patient's request for a transplant because they believe disabled patients may not be able to carry out the complicated medication regimen that organ recipients must adhere to for their entire lives. However, people with disabilities who might have trouble complying with a medication regimen usually have caregivers who can help them with it. Some professionals also believe that, given the scarcity of organs, the available organs should be used for nondisabled people.

Either of these reasons for denying a place on the transplant list is technically illegal. It's discrimination, which is prohibited by federal law. But, the federal laws aren't always enforced. It's up to the patients or their families to point out discrimination when it occurs, which can be a daunting and time-consuming process. To help combat this issue, a number of states have passed state-level laws prohibiting discrimination against people with disabilities with regard to transplant lists.

bioprinting, which is using a specialized 3D printer to create biological structures.

The 3D printer itself is relatively easy to come by—they are expensive but obtainable. The trickier part is the "ink." Obviously, to create an organ that could, in theory, function in a human body, scientists needed to create some sort of biological "ink."

In 2016, scientists Erik Gatenholm and Héctor Martínez Avila worked together to start CELLINK, a company that manufactures bioink made from a seaweed extract. The entrepreneurs expect that bioprinting will start with printing simple tissues like skin or cartilage, but they envision the eventual possibility of printing complex organs like hearts, livers, and kidneys to be used in human transplants. These organs are difficult to print because of their complexity. The heart, for example, has many tiny capillaries that are nearly impossible to print because they are so small.

CELLINK isn't the only company experimenting with bioprinting now, but it has gained much attention in the field because of the promise its bioink product holds. Skeptics of the technology, though, think it may be the stuff of science fiction, and some argue that even if the technology could be developed, it would be so costly that few people could afford it.

Life Support for Organs

Another development that should lead to greater overall success with organ transplants in the future is the TransMedics Organ Care System. This system is essentially a life-support box for organs. Previously, donated organs were transferred to the receiving facility on ice. However, simulating a living environment for the organs keeps them warm and can triple the time window that transplant teams have for getting an organ from donor to recipient. For example, hearts transferred on ice typically have about a four-hour window from removal from the donor to transplant into the recipient. Using the Organ Care System, though, that window is expanded to about twelve hours.

The technology is already being used in the United Kingdom and Australia, and it is in trials in the United States.

Animal-Human Hybrids

In 2018, researchers at Stanford University announced that they had successfully created the first human-sheep hybrids. These hybrids are more than 99 percent sheep, but they have a small number of human stem cells in them.

Scientists believe that this could have a significant impact on the field of organ transplantation. They could technically grow adult-sized organs in about nine months, depending on the animal used. They theorize that for such a xenotransplantation to work, a minimum of 1 percent of the hybrid cells must be human. In theory, they could create such human-sheep hybrids for the sole purpose of obtaining organs needed for transplant.

This has, probably not surprisingly, been met with some backlash. Animal-rights activists argue that it's cruel to animals. Others argue that if the human cells go to the brain of the human-sheep hybrid, then it would

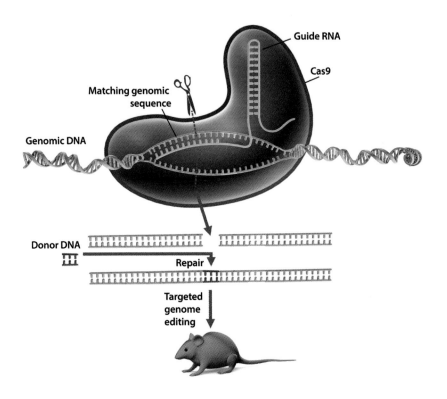

Gene editing could potentially create human-animal hybrids that might hold promise for the future of organ transplantation.

be unethical to kill the animal for the purpose of using its organs.

However, if the ethical issues can be resolved, the technology shows promise. The scientists at Stanford University have already successfully created a mouse pancreas in a rat, which was then transplanted into a diabetic mouse and nearly cured the diabetes.

Artificial Organs

While not currently a viable option for permanent survival, scientists are having some success developing artificial organs that can be used on a temporary basis to keep patients alive while they wait for a transplant. For example, SynCardia Systems has created a fully functioning artificial heart that replaces both heart ventricles and all four heart valves. Heart patients have been kept alive as long as four years while using this device, called the Total Artificial Heart (TAH). Researchers at the University of California, San Francisco have been working on an artificial kidney that can function similarly for patients experiencing kidney failure.

A New Type of Immunotherapy

Scientists are trying a new method of therapy to prevent rejection: transplanting bone marrow along with organs. To do so, the scientists shut down the patient's immune system by destroying the person's T cells. Then, they transplant bone marrow along with the organ in question. (They've begun by experimenting with kidney transplant patients.) The idea is that the transplanted bone marrow tricks the patient's immune system into thinking the transplanted organ is not a foreign invader. The procedure showed some promise when first tried in 2008, and further experimentation is being done to see whether it's a viable therapy.

Xenotransplantation

In some ways pigs hold the most promise for the future of xenotransplantation. Xenotransplantation is the process of grafting or transplanting organs or tissues between members of different species. Pig organs are generally of similar size to adult human organs, and doctors have already found much success in using pig tissue to create human heart valves. This will increase the number of available organs for people who need them.

However, there has been concern about pig tissue potentially carrying viruses that could be transmitted to humans. A recent development in gene editing, though, holds significant potential for the future of pig-human xenotransplantation.

A group of scientists has developed a technology called CRISPR (pronounced "crisper"), which stands for clustered regularly interspaced short palindromic repeats. This technology isolates a protein called Cas9 on the bacterial DNA sequence. It can effectively work like a pair of gene scissors, snipping out segments of DNA from viruses. Using this technology, scientists will no doubt transform the field of organ transplantation.

Using the CRISPR technology, another group of scientists has discovered a way to genetically engineer, or modify, healthy pigs that show no trace of the porcine viruses that could in theory make pig-human transplants unsafe.

Even with this technology, there are still significant obstacles. The human body will still reject the pig organ because it is considered a foreign invader. But rejection is a problem that has been dealt with for years in allotransplants, so in theory, it can eventually be handled in xenotransplantation as well. Removing the danger of porcine virus transmission is a huge step forward in the future of xenotransplantation.

No doubt as scientific discovery continues and the fields of genetics, gene editing, transplantation, and immunosuppression continue to develop, organ transplantation will become more and more successful, leading to many more lives saved. It's anyone's best guess what the future will hold. New discoveries are always on the horizon, and it's just a matter of finding creative ways to solve today's health problems.

Chronology

1823 The first successful skin graft is performed by Dr. Carl Bunger.

1883 The first successful thyroid transplant is performed by Dr. Theodor Kocher.

1902 French surgeon Alexis Carrel begins transplant experiments on dogs, leading to the discovery of organ rejection.

1905 The first successful human cornea transplant is performed by D. Eduard Zirm in what is now the Czech Republic.

1933 Ukrainian surgeon Yurii Voronoy performs the first cadaver-to-living-human kidney transplant. Unfortunately, it failed.

1950 The first kidney transplant is performed by Dr. Richard Lawler in Chicago. It failed ten months later.

1953   The cardiopulmonary bypass pump, or heart-lung machine, is first used successfully in heart surgery.

1954   The first successful living-related kidney transplant is performed by Dr. Joseph Murray at Brigham Hospital, in Boston.

1962   The first successful kidney transplant from a deceased donor is performed by Dr. Joseph Murray and Dr. David Hume at Brigham Hospital.

1963   The first successful lung transplant is performed by Dr. James Hardy at the University of Mississippi Medical Center, in Jackson. The patient lived just eighteen days.

1964   Dr. James Hardy performs both the world's first heart transplant and the world's first heart xenotransplantation by transplanting a chimpanzee heart into a dying human. The heart beat for an hour before stopping.

1966   The first successful kidney-pancreas transplant is performed by Dr. Richard Lillehei and Dr. William Kelly at the University of Minnesota, Twin Cities.

1967   The first successful heart transplant is performed by Dr. Christiaan Barnard at Groote Schuur Hospital, in South Africa.

1968   The first successful heart transplant in the United States is performed by Dr. Norman Shumway at Stanford University Hospital, in Stanford, California.

1981   The first successful heart-lung transplant is performed by Dr. Bruce Reitz and Dr. Norman Shumway at Stanford University Hospital.

1983   Cyclosporine, an immunosuppressant, is approved for commercial use. The first successful long-term single-lung transplant is performed by Dr. Joel Cooper at Toronto General Hospital, in Ontario, Canada.

1984   Baby Fae becomes the first infant subject of a xenotransplantation when she receives the heart of a baboon. She lived one month after the procedure.

1986   The first successful long-term double-lung transplant is performed by Dr. Joel Cooper at Toronto General Hospital.

1989   The first successful segment liver transplant is performed by Dr. Christoph Broelsch at the University of Chicago Medical Center.

1990   The first successful living-related lung transplant is performed by Dr. Vaughn Starnes at Stanford University Medical Center.

1992   The first baboon-to-human liver transplant is performed by Dr. Satoru Todo, Dr. Andreas Tzakis, and Dr. John Fung, working under Dr. Thomas Starzl, at the University of Pittsburgh Medical Center. The recipient, a thirty-five-year-old man, died just over two months later.

1995   The first living-donor kidney is removed using laparoscopic surgery, which made recovery much easier than it was previously for the donor.

1998   The first successful hand transplant is performed by Dr. Earl Owen and Dr. Jean-Michel Dubernard in France.

2005   The first successful partial face transplant is performed by Dr. Bernard Devauchelle and Dr. Jean-Michel Dubernard in France.

2010   The first full-face transplant is performed in Spain by a team of thirty doctors.

2012   CRISPR researchers release their findings that CRISPR/Cas9 technology can be used for gene editing. This is considered one of the most important discoveries in the history of biology, with positive implications for the future of organ transplantation.

Glossary

advance directive A written statement of a person's wishes regarding medical treatment, in case he or she is unable to communicate them.

agglutinate To stick together in a mass.

alveoli Tiny air sacs in the lungs where air is exchanged.

antigen A foreign substance that produces an immune response in the body.

apartheid A system of segregation based on race.

aseptic Free from contamination by bacteria, viruses, or microorganisms.

autoimmune Describes a disease caused by an immune response to substances naturally present in the body.

calcineurin A protein phosphatase that activates the T cells of the immune system.

chromosome A threadlike structure containing genetic material that is found in the nucleus of most living cells.

cirrhosis A complication of liver disease that involves loss of liver cells and irreversible scarring of the liver.

connective tissue Tissue that is found between other tissues in the body.

cornea The transparent layer on the front of the eye.

dialysis A system of purifying blood in place of normal kidney function.

embryonic stem cells Stem cells found in a developing embryo.

exocrine Glands that secrete substances onto a tissue, rather than into the bloodstream.

glucose Blood sugar.

granuloma A mass of granular tissue that forms in response to infection or inflammation.

hemorrhage Excessive blood loss.

immunology The branch of medicine concerning immunity.

ischemia Inadequate blood flow to an organ, such as the heart.

lupus An autoimmune disease that commonly attacks, among other organs, the kidneys.

metabolic disease A condition in which abnormal chemical reactions in the body alter the normal metabolic process.

metabolism The chemical processes necessary to maintain life.

molecule A group of atoms bonded together.

monoclonal antibody An antibody produced by a single clone of cells or cell line and consisting of identical antibody molecules.

nucleotide The basic structural unit of a nucleic acid, such as DNA.

pancreatitis Inflammation of the pancreas.

perfusion To supply an organ with blood or other fluid necessary for life.

polyclonal antibody An antibody that is secreted by different B cell lineages within the body (whereas monoclonal antibodies come from a single cell lineage).

sleep apnea Temporary cessation of breathing during sleep.

stem cell An undifferentiated cell that can turn into more differentiated cells.

streptococcal A type of bacterial infection.

T cell A lymphocyte that participates in the body's immune response.

thyroidectomy Removal of the thyroid gland.

toxicity The quality of being toxic.

vital organs The main organs inside the body, such as the heart, lungs, and brain, that are necessary for life.

xenotransplantation The transplantation of an organ or tissue between two different species.

Further Information

BOOKS

Foran, Racquel. *Organ Transplants*. North Mankato, MN: Essential Library, 2013.

Ignotofsky, Rachel. *Women in Science: 50 Fearless Pioneers Who Changed the World*. San Francisco, CA: Ten Speed Press, 2016.

Latta, Susan M. *Bold Woman of Medicine: 21 Stories of Astounding Discoveries, Daring Surgeries, and Healing Breakthroughs*. Chicago, IL: Chicago Review Press, 2017.

Noyce, Pendred. *Magnificent Minds: 16 Pioneering Women in Science and Medicine*. Boston, MA: Tumblehome Learning, Inc., 2016.

Rogers, Kara. *The Kidneys and the Renal System*. New York, NY: Britannica Educational Publishing, 2011.

WEBSITES

MedlinePlus

https://medlineplus.gov/organtransplantation.html

MedlinePlus is an official government website hosted by the United States National Library of Medicine. It contains a comprehensive overview of organ transplantation with many useful links.

OrganDonor.gov

https://organdonor.gov/about/process/transplant-process.html

Established by the United States Department of Health and Human Services, this website offers organ transplantation statistics and stories. This is also where you can sign up to be an organ donor.

UNOS

https://unos.org

The official website of the United Network for Organ Sharing (UNOS) has a lot of interesting information about organ transplants in the United States, including very current statistics.

World Health Organization

http://www.who.int/transplantation/organ/en/

For a more global look at organ transplants, the World Health Organization (WHO) has a simple but informative website.

Bibliography

Altman, Lawrence. "First Human to Get Baboon Liver Is Said to Be Alert and Doing Well." *New York Times*, June 30, 1992. http://www.nytimes.com/1992/06/30/health/first-human-to-get-baboon-liver-is-said-to-be-alert-and-doing-well.html.

Ansari, Azadeh, and Sandrine Amiel. "First Face Transplant Patient, Isabelle Dinoire, Dies at 49." CNN Health, September 7, 2016. http://www.cnn.com/2016/09/06/health/france-face-transplant-patient-dies/index.html.

Bennett, Abbie. "Surgeon Who Performed Live-Saving Operation on Jimmy Kimmel's Son Graduated from UNC." *News & Observer*, May 7, 2017. http://www.newsobserver.com/news/business/health-care/article149145164.html.

"Breakthrough in Fibrotic Diseases That Cause Organ Failure." ScienceDaily, November 13, 2017. https://www.sciencedaily.com/releases/2017/11/171113123655.htm.

Bresnahan, Samantha. "TransMedics Device Keeps Organs Alive Outside the Body." CNN Health, June 10, 2016. https://edition.cnn.com/2016/06/10/health/transmedics-organs-box-vs.

Brusco, Sam. "MedTech Memoirs: Skin Transplants." Medical Design Technology, May 27, 2015. https://www.mdtmag.com/blog/2015/05/medtech-memoirs-skin-transplants.

"Cirrhosis." Mayo Clinic, accessed March 2, 2018. https://www.mayoclinic.org/diseases-conditions/cirrhosis/symptoms-causes/syc-20351487.

"Cornea Transplant." NHS Choices, May 15, 2015. https://www.nhs.uk/conditions/cornea-transplant/why-its-done/.

"Data." UNOS, February 20, 2018. https://unos.org/data/.

"Dirk van Zyl, 68; Had '71 Transplant." New York Times, July 7, 1994. http://www.nytimes.com/1994/07/07/obituaries/dirk-van-zyl-68-had-71-transplant.html.

"Donation Process." Center for Organ Recovery and Education, accessed March 2, 2018. https://www.core.org/understanding-donation/donation-process.

"Glomerular Diseases." National Institute of Diabetes and Digestive and Kidney Diseases, accessed March 2, 2018. https://www.niddk.nih.gov/health-information/kidney-disease/glomerular-diseases.

"History." Organ Procurement and Transplantation Network, accessed March 2, 2018. https://optn.transplant.hrsa.gov/learn/about-transplantation/history.

"The History of Diabetes." Diabetes Health, January 1, 2015. https://www.diabeteshealth.com/the-history-of-diabetes.

"How Technology Is Changing the Future of Organ Transplants." Orgamites, October 12, 2016. http://orgamites.com/technology-changing-future-organ-transplants.

"Immunosuppressants." National Kidney Foundation, accessed March 2, 2018. https://www.kidney.org/atoz/content/immuno.

Kim, Eun Kyung. "Selena Gomez's Kidney Transplant a Common Risk with Lupus." NBC News, September 14, 2017. https://www.nbcnews.com/health/womens-health/selena-gomez-reveals-secret-kidney-transplant-due-lupus-n801281.

Laurence, Jeremy. "60 Lives Linked in Kidney Donor Chain." *Northern Star*, February 27, 2012. https://www.northernstar.com.au/news/60-lives-linked-kidney-donor-chain/1285131.

Lewis, Tim. "Could 3D Printing Solve the Organ Transplant Shortage?" *Guardian*, July 30, 2017. https://www.theguardian.com/technology/2017/jul/30/will-3d-printing-solve-the-organ-transplant-shortage.

Majno, Guido. "The Ancient Riddle of Sepsis." *Journal of Infectious Diseases* 163 (May 1991): 937–45.

"Mayo Clinic Performs First 'Domino' Transplant in Arizona; Rare Procedure Saves Two Lives at Once, Optimizing Organ Supply." Mayo Clinic, January 28, 2003. https://web.archive.org/web/20030220000729/http://www.mayoclinic.org/news2003-sct/1622.html.

"New Liver for Stormie Jones." *New York Times*, February 20, 1990. http://www.nytimes.com/1990/02/20/science/new-liver-for-stormie-jones.html.

"Nondiscrimination in Organ Transplantation Laws and Toolkit." National Down Syndrome Society, Accessed March 2, 2018. https://www.ndss.org/advocate/ndss-legislative-agenda/healthcare-research/nondiscrimination-in-organ-transplantation-laws-toolkit.

"Organ Transplant and Rejection." Lumen Microbiology, accessed March 2, 2018. https://courses.lumenlearning. com/microbiology/chapter/organ-transplantation-and-rejection.

"Organ Transplants for People with Disabilities: Know Your Rights!" Autistic Self Advocacy Network, accessed March 2, 2018. https://autisticadvocacy.org/wp-content/uploads/2014/03/OrganTransplantationKnowYourRights_final.pdf.

Ossola, Alexandra. "Scientists Grow Full-Sized, Beating Human Hearts from Stem Cells." *Popular Science*, March 16, 2016. https://www.popsci.com/scientists-grow-transplantable-hearts-with-stem-cells.

Redman, Emily. "To Save His Dying Sister-in-Law, Charles Lindberg Invented a Medical Device." Smithsonian. com, September 9, 2015. https://www.smithsonianmag. com/smithsonian-institution/save-his-dying-sister-law-charles-lindbergh-Invented-medical-device-180956526.

Sadowsky, Jeffrey. "How Organ Size Affects the Organ Donation Process." Orlando Health, April 15, 2016. https://www.orlandohealth.com/blog/how-organ-size-affects-the-organ-donation-process.

"Sheep-Human Hybrids Pave the Future for Organ
Transplants: Scientists." Channel News Asia, February
20, 2018. https://www.channelnewsasia.com/news/
health/sheep-human-hybrids-pave-the-future-for-organ-
transplants-9972158.

Sifferlin, Alexandra. "5 Discoveries That Will Change the Future
of Organ Transplants." *Time*, June 6, 2013. http://healthland.
time.com/2013/06/06/5-discoveries-that-will-change-the-
future-of-organ-transplants/slide/artificial-organs.

"Timeline of Historical Events and Significant Milestones."
United States Government Information on Organ Donation
and Transplantation, accessed March 2, 2018. https://
organdonor.gov/about/facts-terms/history.html.

"Types of Replacement Heart Valves." American
Heart Association, accessed March 2, 2018. http://
www.heart.org/HEARTORG/Conditions/More/
HeartValveProblemsandDisease/Types-of-Replacement-
Heart-Valves_UCM_451175_Article.jsp#.Woc3d2bMzm0.

"What Causes Organ Failure?" University of Michigan
Transplant Center, accessed March 2, 2018. http://www.
transweb.org/faq/q32.shtml.

Wood, John W. "Hepatitis A." Austin Community College,
accessed March 2, 2018. http://www.austincc.edu/
microbio/2993p/hav.htm.

Page numbers in **boldface** are illustrations.

Owen, Earl, 68, 84

pancreas
  diabetes and, 12, 21–22, 32,
    34
  failure of, 21–22
  transplant, 22, 32, 33–34, 42,
    58, 63, 75, 82, 93–94
perfusion pump/machines, 9,
  48, 50–51
pig heart/tissue, 74–75, **74**,
  106–107
pulmonary fibrosis, 18–19
pulmonary hypertension,
  18–19

Reitz, Bruce, 61–62, 82–83
rotationplasty, 73
Royal, Coena, **88**
Russell, John, 54–55

sarcoidosis, 18–19
sepsis, 15–16, 23
Shumway, Norman, 61–63,
  82–83
skin graft, 6, **26**, 28–29, 72, 81
Stanford University, 61–63, 105
Starnes, Vaughn A., 65, 84
Starzl, Thomas, 55–58, **56**, 82
stem cells, 7, 40–42, 64, 72–73,
  82, 97–99, **98**

systemic inflammatory
  response syndrome (SIRS),
  23

Thomas, Edward Donnall, 64,
  82
3D organs, printing, 99–102
thyroid, **38**
  transplant, 28, 39, 81
Todo, Satoru, 66
TransMedics Organ Care
  System, 102–103
transplant centers, 94–95
triangulation, 50
Tzakis, Andreas G., 66

United Network for Organ
  Sharing (UNOS), 91–94,
  100

Voronoy, Yurii, 29

waiting lists for organs, 7, 35,
  47, 76–78, 93–94, 100–101

xenotransplants, 55, 66–68,
  74–75, 82–83, 103–107

Zirm, Eduard, 81

About the Author

Cathleen Small is the author of dozens of educational books. She has written on everything from history to biography to science and enjoys the wide range of topics she gets to explore on a daily basis. When she's not writing or editing, Small enjoys traveling and spending time with her family. She resides in the San Francisco Bay Area with her husband, who works in the biotech industry, and their two sons.